WOMEN & FOOD

Tabitha Hume RDSA
with
Dr Dora Wynchank FC Psych

ZEBRA

Published by Zebra Press, a division of
the Struik New Holland Publishing Group (Pty) Ltd
80 McKenzie Street
Cape Town 8001
South Africa

First edition, first impression October 2000
Copyright © in published edition Zebra Press 2000
Text © Tabitha Hume 2000
'Dr Dora' boxes and chapter 13 © Dora Wynchank 2000

10 9 8 7 6 5 4 3 2 1

Managing editor Frances Perryer
Copy editors Delene Slabbert and Frances Perryer
Cover concept Jonathan Edwards
Cover design Jonathan Edwards and Christian Jaggers
Book design Crazy Cats and B-Complex
DTP B-Complex

Cover reproduction by Hirt & Carter Cape (Pty) Ltd
Reproduction by Trident Press (Pty) Ltd
Printed and bound by Trident Press (Pty) Ltd

ISBN 1 86872 357 7

CONTENTS

FOREWORD

Depression is an extremely common illness, and can strike as many as 15% of the population at some stage in their lives. It is roughly twice to three times as common in females as males, although the reason for this is not clear. It is possible that this difference relates to societal role and identity issues, or it may relate to innate biological differences that are poorly understood.

What is increasingly overwhelmingly demonstrated by recent research advances is that depression is a disease, with measurable changes in a vast number of areas. Perhaps the most important are alterations in the brain's chemical transmitter systems, and a huge body of literature exists documenting these changes in a large number of neurotransmitters. In addition, changes in brain metabolism and blood flow patterns have been replicated in many studies. These changes tend to reverse on successful treatment. It is part of folklore that 'you are run down, that's why you have caught the bug'; new research unequivocally shows that one's immune system is altered in depression.

All this hard evidence that depression is a disease stands in stark contrast to the fact that it remains poorly understood and stigmatised. Employers are far less likely to give an employee with depression the same leeway as they would with ordinary physical illness. The stigma extends to the medical aid and insurance industries, where equitable resources for treatment are often not afforded to people with depression. Lastly, friends and family may aggravate the problem by less than sage advice. Urging a sufferer to snap out of it or feeding them sensationalistic stories about the dangers of treatment are common scenarios.

Depression is often difficult to diagnose in the community. Less than 25% of depressed patients are diagnosed and treated in American studies, and the likelihood is that this figure may be worse in more poorly resourced settings. This may be due to inadequate time in the average primary care consultation, lack of awareness of the typical diagnostic symptoms of mood disorder, or failure of patients to recognise and report their physical symptoms as being associated with depression. A substantial problem remains the significant stigma attached to diagnoses of psychiatric illness in general and depression in particular. There is a regrettably held belief that depression is self induced and that it can be managed by simply encouraging patients to pull themselves together. Understanding that depression is a clinical disorder with a neurochemical basis that is easily treatable is not widespread. Many patients with depression would rather have a physical than a psychiatric diagnosis. Cultural factors are also important and there is a tendency to under-diagnose psychiatric illness, particularly depression, in a cross cultural setting.

The symptoms of depression are associated with significant complications. Loss of interest in leisure activities is almost universal, together with a change in eating habits. People struggle to cope at their previous level in their work, and absenteeism and poor productivity are common problems. Relationships often suffer, as the person is irritable, negative, withdrawn and tends to lose interest in sex. In more severe depression, life becomes meaningless, and people see death as the only solution to their distress. Suicide is the most dramatic and tragic complication of depression.

With modern treatments the management of depression is a rewarding exercise. The vast majority of depressed patients are able to be dramatically and effectively treated. This simplicity of treatment needs to be seen in context of the fact that depression is a severely incapacitating disorder with significant risks to the patient. Modern approaches to treatment are effective and if used judiciously, relatively free of significant problems.

In this book the picture of depression is elegantly and skilfully depicted. The book interweaves valuable clinical insights into a scientific framework, making this complex and important subject both accessible and entertaining. It is a valuable resource, taking a different angle to this prevalent and currently under-developed area.

Michael Berk
Associate Professor
Department of Psychiatry
Wits Medical School

WHY A PSYCHIATRIST CONTRIBUTED TO THIS BOOK

You may be wondering why on earth a psychiatrist is participating in a 'diet book'. Well, this is a book about women, food and mood; and I am fascinated by all three areas. I am a doctor specialising both in mental illness and mental health. For several years now, I have been trying to unravel the relationship between women, their bodies and their minds. I feel passionately about women's issues in all areas, but particularly in my field of work. The position of women has hit the forefront of politics; it's about time that it surfaced in medicine too!

Indeed, women have always had an ambivalent relationship with mental health professionals. For at least four centuries, more women than men have been diagnosed with mental illness. By the 17th century, twice as many cases of insanity were reported amongst women as compared to men. By the 19th century, most people in 'lunatic asylums' were women, from all social classes.

On the one hand, all women were considered mentally weak, frivolous and unstable. They were vulnerable to episodes of hysteria and were certainly not be trusted with the vote. On the other hand, it was not considered 'ladylike' to suffer from mental illness. So what could a woman do? The founder of an esteemed medical journal, the *British Journal of Psychiatry*, warned in 1853 that 'if insanity is a disease requiring medical treatment, ladies cannot legally or properly undertake [that] treatment' (quoted by H Crimlisk and S Welch in an essay, 'Women and Psychiatry', in the same journal [no. 169, pp.6-9] in 1996).

Not much has changed. Even today, we know that women tend to be the majority of psychiatric patients. They are also more likely than men to receive prescriptions for psychiatric medication. Yet until 1993, women were barred from research studies for new drugs in the United States. Only men took part in these studies. So, treatments that were developed before 1993 were never tested on women! Exactly how the drugs work in women's bodies has only been examined recently.

It is true that certain mental illnesses are far more common in women than in men. Depression occurs about twice as often in women and anxiety disorders affect women three times as often as men. These findings emerge consistently in study after study, regardless of social class, ethnic group or country of origin. Why is this so? I attempt to address the facts and fallacies of women's mental health throughout the book.

Turning our attention to women and food, we find as much controversy. Any women's magazine illustrates this relationship beautifully. In the first part of the magazine we see youthful, skinny models and wish we could shed a few kilos to look as good. Week after week, we read articles with tips on optimum weight loss; but nothing seems to work. Then we page on to the culinary section to find mouth-watering recipes with luscious photographs. What mixed messages! As women, we are expected to nurture everyone else. We excel at preparing food and yet we feel guilty if we 'indulge' ourselves in eating. How can we look eternally young, svelte and attractive as well as enjoy our own cooking? This is a quandary that is difficult to resolve. Perhaps it contributes to the development of eating disorders, so common in society. Even if women do not have full-blown anorexia or bulimia, they often have a lifelong, fraught and ambivalent relationship with food. I explore the connection between women's eating patterns and their brain chemicals, in an attempt to shed some light on this field.

This brings me to my third area of interest: neurochemistry. As a psychiatrist, I am in the privileged position of having studied the workings of the brain from both a psychological and a biological perspective. The brain controls and determines everything about us, from thinking to dreaming to behaviour – yet, its workings remained a mystery until very recently. In many ways, the brain is still our most elusive organ.

However, the mystery is beginning to be understood. Throughout the world, neuroscientists are devoting themselves to the study of the brain and mental illness. There is new hope for conditions that were previously considered to be incurable. Amongst all fields of medical research, I believe that understanding brain function is the most exciting and rapidly expanding. Unfortunately, very few people keep up to date with the advances in brain research. They switch off when brain function is mentioned because they feel that it is far too difficult to understand. Sure, it is complicated, but not impossible to comprehend. I have illustrated some of these findings in a simplified way, for everyone to learn. You will notice as you read my contribution, which is easily identifiable in boxes, that scientific articles or books have been referenced with a number. If you page to the References section at the back of the book, you will find the names of the journals and other publications listed in full. Of course, I am aware of the danger involved in radical simplification. The real meaning of complex issues may get lost in the attempt to explain. Where there is uncertainty or controversy, I indicate so in my text. But you will experience the latest research findings as literally mind boggling!

I would like to invite you to learn more about these discoveries. Let me challenge the way you have thought of emotion, mental illness and appetite. You will find that the more you learn, the more you want to discover and the more questions you will ask. It can be hard to keep up with the advance in knowledge. My contribution to this book is an attempt to bring you up to date with the cutting edge of neuroscience in a way that is easy to understand. I hope you have as much fun in the reading as I did in the writing!

Dora Wynchank
Johannesburg, August 2000

WHY I WROTE
THIS BOOK

Obesity has now become a problem of global proportions. It is an epidemic, spanning countries, populations, creeds and social backgrounds alike. But we dieticians at The X Clinics do not only treat clinical obesity and Syndrome X. We also treat a range of other diseases, as well as people who are not overweight, but are terrified of that prospect.

As a result of this fear of obesity and overweight, the media and the public alike have moved into an era focused on aesthetics, whereby 'nice and thin' has become an all-consuming obsession. To be thin is to be nice. To be thin is to be successful. And to be thin is to be happy.

This skin-deep fixation has led not only to the emergence of problems such as anorexia and bulimia nervosa, but also to what we call dysfunctional eating. The fear of food people have developed has replaced the age-old culinary passions which originally gave food its rightful position in the hearts of families, lovers and religions.

Misconceptions about dieting and losing weight (a term banished in our clinics) have incorrectly led people to calorie-cutting and starvation, which wreak havoc with the body and brain alike. Recent studies have now linked the occurrence of fad dieting and clinical depression, leading to the realisation that there is much deeper damage done by such dieting methods. In fact, many people who come to The X Clinics present with underlying depressive symptoms which have been precipitated by fad dieting and severe calorie cutting.

Most people who have gained weight want a quick fix, and so will try literally anything (and spend literally anything) to lose weight and become 'acceptable' again. The best way to achieve this seems to be to eat less, or even stop eating. Even a medical practitioner who was unaware of the work I was doing in the clinic laughed one evening, 'Come on! The best way to lose weight is to stop eating for a while!'

The problem is, it works! It works immediately, and is almost fool-proof in its effectiveness. But at last, the public are beginning to wake up to the truth: dieting doesn't work in the long-term. Inevitably, the weight gets put on again, along with newly acquired food obsessions, dysfunctional eating, and an increased sense of being out of control of the body. This leads to 'trying nearly every diet that exists', and repeated losses, each time gaining to a greater weight than before.

Each time, however, the brain is affected, bit by bit, eventually leading to a long-term alteration in not only thought processes, but also chemical functioning. This descent into varying degrees of psychiatric disease has made simple dietetic practice frustratingly complicated, and has led us to delve further into what actually happens with each dramatic weight loss attempt – and the findings are not positive. Although it is not quite as simple as saying that dieting leads to clinical depression, the correlations are staggering – and this is why I am writing this book.

Depression can be brought about by continuous dieting, but it can also be hereditary or brought on by life circumstances such as severe and ongoing stress and anxiety. Whatever the reason for the depression, the problem initiates or exacerbates body fat gain. The reasons for this will be highlighted in this book. An individual who has never before had had a fat problem may develop one as a result of depression. 'Comfort eating' actually only plays a small part in this physical change, the main reasons not being psychological, but rather a complete alteration in the body's metabolic functioning, leading to unexplained weight problems.

When people begin the therapy we prescribe for them, we often find that their progress is slower than we, or they, had anticipated. Delving further into the patient's physiological make-up, however, often leads to the diagnosis of underlying psychiatric disorders such as clinical depression. The physical side-effects of depression are actually the reason for their bodies not losing fat as expected. Unfortunately, the ignorant public stigma associated with such conditions often leads to an immediate block against acknowledgement and treatment of the disorder, which would otherwise lead to healthy fat loss, associated with a healthy body. The patient's response to such a diagnosis and treatment is usually hostile and defensive, and thus treatment of this preventing factor is halted, with frustrating consequences to the patient and practitioner.

Unfortunately, if the underlying depression is not treated, the only other way to lose fat is to further restrict calories, and enter deeper and deeper into the problem. This foolproof starvation regimen is what I nick-name 'the override button' approach to weight loss: despite what the reasons for the overweight may be, and despite what damage it does to the body, it will work. You will lose weight by starving. But so will you lose weight by cutting off three of your limbs.

We are interested in treating the body, not just in getting a result. After all, the reason for a change in the make-up of the body is an imbalance of something: and it is not always food at all!

I share this frustration with my colleagues in the clinics. Our struggle to enable people to be healed of their other problems before healthy fat loss can occur prompted me to write this book We desperately need to explain away the fears associated with psychiatric disease, so that we can dietetically treat a healthy body, not merely guarantee an 'override button' fat loss, regardless of the reasons or consequences.

Due to the overwhelming presence of such issues in our day-to-day dealings with patients, our interest in basic psychiatry has, to a large extent, helped us de-stigmatise depression and psychiatric disorders. We have found it exceptionally useful to speak in a down-to-earth manner, explaining this previously fearful subject in the same light-hearted manner as we do other physical problems. It is as such that I write this book.

The success of **The X Diet** as a widespread educational tool to remove the confusion associated with weight control has given me 'poetic' licence to continue in the same style of writing. I been grateful to receive comments from many readers about how they could 'hear' me talking to them in previous books. Thus, I have satisfied my goal: to literally chat to the reader and share my passion for learning. I write as I speak, and I speak as I think. Devoid of flowery prose, I wish to teach and share what I know.

I hope this book will be a fun and enlightening journey of discovery into the complexities of how food and the mind interact, so as to gain a non-threatening view of very common disorders. It does not pretend to be a literary prize-winner, but I hope it will help to elucidate how real these problems are, and bring many more people to a healthy way of life.

Tabitha Hume
The X Clinic, Johannesburg
(011) 788 7625
Cape Town: (021) 465 8114/5/7/9
Durban: (031) 764 1969

Acknowledgements

Writing this book has certainly been filled with hardships; time changes, excitement of coinciding with the opening of our Durban and new Cape Town branches, and many more exciting new findings on the dietetics front, which has meant adding and adjusting the original draft to try and keep up with the latest research findings.

This turmoil is exactly what makes life wonderful, diverse and exceptionally challenging. And it is exactly that: life! However, I have been exceptionally lucky to be surrounded by a team consisting of superb people, who have contributed to this book, and whom I would like to thank:

To Dora Wynchank, for her invaluable contribution to the book; to Professor Michael Berk, for doing me the great honour of writing a foreword, and to Vitalab for their contribution on polycystic ovarian syndrome.

To my colleagues at the clinics, Nicole Sacks, Shona Vlaming, Nikki Lee Hirschson, Patricia Hoar, and our newest associates, Justine Aginsky and Sarah Wildy, whose abilities to hold the fort while 'the book' was taking over, have helped make it a reality.

To my mother, Toni Hume, whose unending support both as a friend, mother and queen of organising, has helped pull everything together and keep it going. I hope to receive some of your genes, at least.

To Jonathan Edwards, my brother in law, whose magnificent artistic talent has turned thought into visual explanation.

To my other friends and relatives who have put up with me, and given excellent criticism along the way and at the final hour, when the final proof went in: Sarah Hume, Carol Hathorn and Lisa Hall, who waded through pages of proof and gave an 'outsider's' view.

To my father, David Hume, who with Jonathan Edwards, created the cover: brainstorming was fun, but I will still never fathom how your brains work!

And finally, to my amazing husband, David Edwards. Some things in life just go right. You are one of those things, and I wish to express that most of my achievements have been made possible by the encouragement, late-night companionship at the computers, and endless patience you have constantly given me.

And for believing in my passion for my work.

As with any big project, there are always others behind the scenes whose contribution is invaluable. I extend a warm thanks to all those people who have also helped to make this possible.

1 THE STIGMA ATTACHED TO CLINICAL DEPRESSION

Misconceptions about clinical depression cause a great deal of hurt to the unfortunate individuals who suffer from this disorder. Often treated in an insensitive way, they are scorned by an ill-informed society.

The following scenario illustrates a paradigm:

A young corporate executive is rushing to work early one morning. She needs to get to the office on time for a very important meeting at nine. The meeting is critical to clinch a major deal that she has been working on for months. However, an unprecedented thunderstorm causes traffic to progress slowly. It's obvious that she will be late for the meeting and feeling increasingly desperate, she calls her secretary from the car to find out if her client has arrived yet. While dodging cars and puddles, she concentrates intensely on the anxiety in her secretary's voice, and fails to see the red light...

As she opens her eyes, her mother hovers tearfully over the bed. Confused, she tries to get up, but realises she can't move her legs. Taking her hand, her mother quietly explains that she was involved in a car accident yesterday. Her spinal cord has been severed and the prognosis is irreversible: she is a paraplegic.

From this moment on, her life changes forever. The most basic tasks now seem impossible. As she moves in society, people see her differently; seeing the wheelchair before they see her. She notices that it is uncomfortable for others to watch her struggle. Some people kindly offer to help; others are awkward around her. But one thing is certain: society accepts her disability. Fate, not her own choice, put her in that chair, and no one questions this.

Even if it had been her fault, people are compassionate. Everyone has done careless things once or twice but most people are lucky. Nobody ever expects such a tragic outcome of events. Why was life so unfair to her?

Do people scorn the paraplegic? Do they consider her 'stupid' because she cannot stand up and reach the top shelf? Or 'lazy' because she won't even try to walk?

These questions should curdle your insides as I ask them because the answers are so blatantly obvious. Society accepts her disability because paraplegia is recognised as a tangible problem for which there is no cure. The paraplegic is no less of a person because she can't use her legs.

Simple. We acknowledge the condition, respect the disability and move on without the slightest question. But clinical depression is another matter altogether!

Let us revisit our stressed executive battling her way through the rain, and change the outcome. This time, there is no accident. She gets to the meeting – albeit late, flustered and breathless. And she clinches the deal. Then, over the next few weeks, for no obvious reason, her career starts disintegrating. She becomes increasingly tearful and cannot cope with tasks that were effortless before. She is dogged by feelings of hopelessness and guilt, and worries continuously. She longs for the oblivion of sleep, but wakes up at 2 am every morning. Daytimes are excruciating; she is constantly exhausted, forgetful and irritable. She starts gaining weight. Nothing gives her pleasure any more. Nothing excites her like it used to. Everything is going so well, why does she feel these things?

Mention that she may have 'depression' and see people's eyes glance sideways and their voices drop. Notice the prejudice in society around mental illness.

'This woman is strange. I mean, she's changed. I just can't be around her any more.'

'How embarrassing! She is unpredictable and out of control, it's just too weird! I don't know anything about that sort of stuff.'

'Some special doctor can deal with her, thank you!'

'Anyway, why doesn't she pull herself together and carry on? I mean, she has everything: a good home, a loving family and a high-powered job. And yet she says she has a problem? Rubbish!'

'She's just too self-indulgent to take the rough with the smooth like the rest of us do. We all have mornings when we battle to get

out of bed. But do we stay there? Never! There is a life to live!'
'And how could she do that to her children and her sweet husband? Putting all that responsibility onto her family and friends! Huh! I would love to be able to do that, but I don't make my problems anyone else's.'
'She must stop feeling so sorry for herself and just get on with it!'

This aggressive sentiment is a fraction of what many ignorant people say about people suffering from depression. I see it almost daily with patients and their husbands, even with their doctors. People who have been diagnosed with depression are shunned by society – a society that seems to have made little progress in this area since the days of burning witches at the stake.

To see how ludicrous it all sounds to the learned mind, place yourself in the mind of the paraplegic one more time, and then 'hear' this paragraph in a different context:
'This woman is strange. I mean, she has changed. I just can't be around her any more – I would feel too embarrassed!'
'I have no idea what she'll do next! Heavens, no! I don't know anything about that sort of stuff! Leave me out of this one! Some special doctor can deal with that, thank you!'
'No, I'm sorry, it's just too strange!' And so on …

And yet this is the way clinical depressives are often treated! This is also what we are trying to change. There must be no more stigmas, no more bias, and no more judgement.

DR DORA: A psychiatrist's view of depression

Clinical depression is a serious disorder with firmly established biological causes. If left untreated, it can take a debilitating course. The outcome may even be death. Few people know that depression is the biggest single risk factor for suicide and that 10% of depressives end up killing themselves. Yet many people in society seem to carry on as if it does not exist. Somehow, if people cannot see the physical damage, they assume that the illness simply does not exist.

How often have you heard, 'it's all in the mind'? But the mind is not just an abstract concept; science is proving that it has a very physical basis. Our society does not keep up with scientific discoveries about depression. So the prejudices remain.

The power of the brain

The brain is a mass of soft, rubbery and yellowish matter, convoluted into various difficult-to-define areas. It is hard to imagine, by just looking at a human brain, how powerful it is, and how much lies within it.

Scientists have tried to unravel its mysteries for ages. The ancient Greeks believed the brain to be the seat of our souls, but not our thoughts. Then it was noted that nerves joined the eyes to this brain, therefore it had to be part of some processing. Various other stepping-stones were laid down (one of the more bizarre of these was phrenology, or mind-mapping from the bumps on the skull), to attempt to define specific areas of individual function. There are ongoing studies to help us understand the brain's functioning more clearly.

'The more is discovered,' wrote pharmacologist and physicist Susan Greenfield, 'the more there is still to learn. It is a little like the monster of Greek mythology, the hydra: once one head was cut off, seven grew in its place.'

No wonder the study of the brain sparks a feeling of unease within, and no wonder many derisively shrug off its anomalies.

DR DORA: Bump-reading the brain, and other historical quirks...

Franz Gall was the founder of phrenology, a pseudoscientific discipline of the 19th century. He proclaimed that bumps on the skull (that can be felt by running your fingers over the scalp) identified all of the areas of the brain that lay below.[1] A large 'love bump' on the back of the skull would predict a person of a very loving disposition. You can imagine the view modern medicine takes of phrenology! But Gall was certainly not the first person to propose a bizarre theory of psychiatry. The brain and its function have baffled thinkers for centuries.

How the mentally ill have been understood and treated has varied greatly from era to era. Tracing this history helps us understand the ethos of the time. The earliest societies understood all disease to be caused by a spiritual battle between good and evil. Mental illness, especially, was attributed to evil spirits. Treatment involved exorcism (which did not always work!) Witchcraft and demonic possession are still considered useful explanations of eccentric behaviour. Many alleged witches who were burnt at the stake probably had some form of mental illness.[2]

In the Babylonian civilisation, medicine and religion were one. Later on, the Greeks proposed a more scientific view of mental illness. The body, brain and soul were all considered important in diagnosis and treatment. In the Middle Ages, once again, religion and mysticism held sway. People who sinned were believed to be punished by mental illness. Even until recently, folklore held that people were especially vulnerable to depression and other mental illness at the time of the new moon. The word 'lunatic' is derived from the Latin for moon. Many studies of the last 20 years have refuted this view.[3-5] There was even a slightly *decreased* rate of absenteeism from the workplace at full moon.[6] The suicide rate in another study was shown to be no different at full moon.[7]

The Renaissance brought a rebirth of the scientific method in studying medicine. The mind was considered 'unscientific' and only philosophers and the clergy dabbled with it. This prejudice persisted until the 19th century. In 1808, the term *psychiatry* was coined and by the end of that century, the fundamentals of psychology had been established.[8] But not only has there been discrimination against the mentally ill, those who work with them have also experienced prejudice (psychiatrists being called 'head shrinkers', for example). As recently as the 1960s, there was a resurgence of 'antipsychiatry' feeling that is still prevalent in certain circles today.[9]

The 20th century brought an appreciation of the complexity of the brain and mind that has exploded in terms of knowledge over the last few decades. The study of the nervous system is called *neuroscience*. Neuroscientists are researchers from different fields who use many techniques to decipher the mystery of the brain. And they are winning. Neuroscience is the most rapidly advancing field in medicine. Every month, new discoveries are made. We are learning more and more about the 'big picture' as well as what happens where even the microscope cannot see. For example, we are getting to understand what each part of the brain does, why things sometimes go wrong and how nerves cells 'talk' to one another. This quest for knowledge is not restricted to the laboratory – even governments are now involved. At the start of 1990, the United States Congress declared that the nineties would be the 'Decade of the Brain'. Millions of dollars were allocated to fund research in neuroscience and we are seeing the results.

Neuroscientists should not ignore social and psychiatric aspects of the human condition. The current emphasis in psychiatric research incorporates all of these disciplines.[10]

Misconceptions about depression

Perhaps we should begin with the common misconceptions people have about depression. From the most extreme perspective, certain people might use a religious framework to explain why people get depressed. They might say that depression is the work of the devil pushing aside all that is good and replacing it with negativity.

While this argument sounds attractively simple, it is simplistic. Firstly, a 'culprit' for the illness has been identified: the devil. But, is depression some agent's fault? Is it judgemental to adopt a blaming attitude? Secondly, the emotions experienced in depression are being confused with a spiritual experience. While it is true that many people suffering from depression describe a kind of heavy, hopeless feeling, is this an emotion or a spiritual battle? People who interpret what happens to them in the light of a religious experience may assume that if 'religion' is the only cause, it must be the only cure. Unfortunately, it is not so simple. Many religious authorities would agree that prayer alone does not cure major depression. Prayer may form part of a holistic treatment package tailored for the individual's needs, but in isolation it can be abused by the mentally ill.

DR DORA: More misconceptions about depression

Some religious groups advocate that their members stop taking psychiatric medication and promise to cure by spiritual means alone. From a psychiatrist's point of view, it is extremely dangerous to deny the physical causes of depression. While alternative methods such as prayer may work for the occasional person, the majority of depressives will sink back into a life-threatening, incapacitating illness.

A second opinion that also attributes blame to the sufferer is that the individual is not trying hard enough to be happy. In this case, depression is understood to be like an ongoing sadness in a person with no will power. This theory is perhaps one of the major contributors to the stigma associated with depression.

Here, the question needs to be asked: is it fair to ask a person suffering from major depression to 'try to be happy'? Once you have read how psychiatrists define a depressive episode – you can decide whether this kind of mood disorder is under voluntary control or not.

DR DORA: What is major depressive disorder?

Briefly stated, psychiatrists define major depressive disorder as an illness where three major aspects of human functioning are affected:

- mood
- physical function
- thinking.

To start with the first area: *mood* is the internal 'emotional climate' of an individual. In major depression, mood is low most of the day, nearly every day. Depressed people are weepy and gloomy. Sometimes they feel 'dead inside'. Things that used to bring them pleasure no longer do so.

Physical functions that are affected in major depression refer to things the body does that we simply take for granted. For example, in the depressed individual, sleep, appetite, sex drive, energy levels and bodily movement are all altered.

Thinking becomes distorted in depression. Both the *way* people think (memory, concentration, decision making) and *what* they think, change. The thought content of the depressive is pessimistic in three ways: self-esteem is shaky, the world outside seems bleak and the future seems unbearable. Thoughts of death commonly recur; guilt feelings predominate and 'the light at the end of the tunnel' is simply invisible.

The episode lasts at least two weeks (often much longer) and causes severe distress. The person's level of functioning declines in every important area: work, social life and leisure.

Another biased viewpoint is that these people are only sad because there is some subconscious reward to be reaped. And there are people who, although they may well have major clinical depression, and need psychiatric care, also have psychological issues to deal with. They need to accept support from people around them and turn to professionals for the correct help, but those around them do not necessarily give them the correct support, and possibly give them too much, thereby 'feeding' the psychological problems being masked by the psychiatric symptoms. Here, I am describing people who always feel that they are the 'victims' of a situation. They complain of being unhappy all of the time. They feel that they are always dealt the 'short straw' and constantly demand pity, attention and concern from others.

These victims may exist in an unhealthy relationship with people around them who assume a 'caregiver' role. The victim often struggles to make decisions independently and needs the assistance of caregivers. Ironically, when responsibility is stripped from the victims their cries of helplessness become a self-fulfilling prophecy. They eventually believe that they are useless. With the rest of the whines comes a very truthful moan, 'I can't even do that by myself!' The straw gets shorter by the day, as does the feeling of loss of control. Finally, they are totally dependent and left with very little self-esteem, which is fundamental to simple human dignity.

'Caregivers' may also have psychological problems. Being needed so desperately props up their own poor self-esteem. This negative mutual reinforcement may eventually result in the caregiver being able to scorn the victim. It may also be difficult for such a caregiver to allow the victim more autonomy. The prospect of the victim taking control and getting better would upset the whole applecart entirely. If the victim is no longer the victim, then who will need the caregiver? But remember that supporting and believing in someone are very different from doing it all for them.

Is the interaction that has been described above an example of depression – or is it a maladaptive personality type? Most psychiatric authorities would recognise this sort of behaviour and attitude as evidence of a dependent personality style.

DR DORA: Dependence and co-dependence

People with dependent personality styles need to be taken care of and are terrified of separation. Typically, they are clingy, submissive and long to please. From a statistical point of view, they are more commonly women than men.[11] The dependent personality may :

- have difficulty making everyday decisions without excessive advice and reassurance from others
- need others to assume responsibility for them
- struggle to express disapproval of others because they might lose support or approval
- find it difficult to initiate projects alone because of their poor self-confidence
- even volunteer to do unpleasant tasks (such as cleaning toilets!) to gain approval from others
- avoid being alone as it is dreadful for them
- hate being single and catapult from one relationship to the next to avoid this
- spend a lot of energy worrying about being left alone.[12]

According to some researchers on the subject of personality type, dependent people avoid harm by worrying about the future. They also depend on rewards, such as the approval of others.[13] These characteristics are believed to be genetically inherited. In fact, much of what constitutes personality is inherited.

What about those people who end up caring for the dependent person? They may also have emotional difficulties such as needing to be needed. This pathological relationship is referred to as co-dependence.

Another misconception is that depressed people can 'snap out of it'. This is the thinking behind, "Oh, just wait until this period of stress is over, it's just a phase". There are two issues here: the first is the relationship between stress and depression. Can severe ongoing stress cause depression? Yes! But it can be so severe, and over such a prolonged time, that the eventual result is physical distress, which is organic or physical in nature, affecting the chemicals in the brain. The second issue is whether or not it is possible for a depressed person to 'snap out of it'. Is depressed mood voluntary? No!

DR DORA: Can the depressed person simply 'snap out of it'?

The quick answer is no. There are several reasons for this which we will explore in some detail. Depression tends to be an ongoing illness. In one large American study, the average duration of a depressive episode was six months.[14] In other words, the nature of the illness is that it goes on and on. It is not short-lived, like a cold. Even after one year of being depressed, 31% of people will *still* be depressed.[15] This finding emerged from a five-year study of 431 subjects.

In order to answer this question, we also have to understand some of the recent findings of neuroanatomists. These researchers try to answer the question: what is happening to the brain of a depressed person that can be observed in the laboratory? Indeed, the brains of depressives behave very differently from those who are not depressed. Amongst other things, depressed people's brains tend to be underactive. Particularly, the area of the brain that controls observation of the outside world is 'turned off'. So simply transplanting a person to another environment will not help.

DR DORA: Stress, depression and illness

Any person who has experienced terrible stress will say it wears you down, psychologically and physically. But can this 'truth' be tested scientifically? One way to check the effects of stress is to measure what it does to cells that help the body to defend itself from infection. These 'soldier' cells are part of the immune system. Indeed, a number of studies have shown that exposure to severe stress tends to suppress the immune response.

It was only as recently as 1975 that two researchers proved that the immune system could be controlled by the mind.[16] In a fascinating experiment, they showed quite by chance that psychological function could control the number of white blood cells produced by the immune system. Since then, it has become firmly established that the brain, hormones and the immune system are linked to and influence each other.

A recent study examined whether stressed people were more likely to develop a common cold. The researchers found that the more stress people reported; the more likely they were to report an infection with one of five different cold viruses.[17]

Enthusiastic researchers often test their hypotheses on medical students, who become the 'guinea pigs' of many different studies. Another study compared exam time, a time of extremely high stress for medical students, to a time of no stress at all. During exam time, the students' immune systems were less active and they tended to suffer from more respiratory infections.[18]

But, the stressed individual is not always a medical student! Another study examined 26 people whose spouses were severely ill. Over time, the caregivers' immune systems deteriorated compared to the control group. This suggests that the longer the duration of the stress, the worse its effect.[19]

Not only does severe stress dampen the immune response: depression and anxiety can also affect the body's ability to defend itself from infection. For example, when a group of research subjects (medical students again!) were exposed to the hepatitis B vaccine, the calmer students mounted a stronger immune reaction than the more anxious students did.[20] Certain lethal cancers are more likely in depressed people, according to another 17 year study.[21]

But not all stress is bad. In fact, mild stress is essential to keep us alert, motivated and to stimulate emotional growth. In another experiment, mild stress was found to boost the defensive response of certain 'soldier cells' of the immune system (natural killer cells and interleukin-2 production).[22]

Ongoing stress can increase cholesterol to above-normal levels. On the other hand, a week in the Bahamas will not prevent a possible heart attack from occurring; the damage has already been done to the heart. There is now a chronic disease that needs ongoing therapy.

The same applies to depression. Stress and pressures of life may be the trigger for depression, but once it is there, it needs a lot more than just a 'break' to sort it out. Before a holiday, you often hear someone saying, 'I can't wait to get away! I can really relax and then come back all fresh and rearing to go.' Then upon return, it takes 24 hours before they feel as pathologically overwhelmed and strife-ridden as before.

The individual will interpret this as an innate inability to cope with life, and develop a low self-esteem; yet another example of how ignorance about depression can leave deep-seated psychological problems in its wake. Ongoing stress can certainly be debilitating, but every so often this stress turns into a more chronic alteration of the functioning of the brain. This is called depression, and if left untreated, can lead to death by either prolonged lifestyle diseases such as heart disease and cancer, or suicide. The sufferer will often deny flatly that s/he cannot cope, nor that s/he is a possible candidate for suicide, but this kind of denial can simply hasten the progression of the disorder towards an unpleasant outcome.

In society today, stress is as common as having a glass of water. In fact, some people pride themselves on being stressed: it shows them to be powerful business people with lots of responsibility, 'making the most out of their lives' and not wasting time. It could also be an expression of loyalty to a company, or a means of 'keeping up with the Joneses'. Parents often talk about their offspring proudly, in tones of, 'He is under so much pressure with this new company' as if his pressure is a yardstick for success.

After all, in this goal-driven world, relaxing with the cat can be viewed as laziness, or holidaying alone, in a remote destination as 'peculiar'. After all, we should be relieving all this 'stress' in yet another stressful environment; one that is filled with cigarette-advert demi-goddesses with Barbie-doll bodies with the well-trained ability to leap on and off water-bikes, accompanied by bronzed Adonises, bodies honed to perfection by hours in the gym which their careers don't even allow for, if they are the same careers that afford them the income necessary to sail yachts at that age!

I think that people misunderstand the saying work hard, play hard. This does not mean play as hard as you work. It means relax hard. Really hard. Like lying down and just dreaming once in a while, without the guilt or fear of being completely alone making you feel uncomfortable. If being alone and quiet does make you feel uneasy, you are doing the right thing by reading this book.

Depression is not a weakness or a sin. It does not mean that you are lazy, and it does not deserve self-hatred or self-belittling to be 'forgiven' for being the person you are. Neither does it require excessive ambition to 'prove' to the world that you are more than what you feel you are. Depression should be treated with the same respect that you would afford a wild animal that threatened your life. But, unfortunately, so few people understand and empathise with this affliction, those who suffer from depression are forced to remain silent about a clinical condition that is viewed as 'shameful', rather than frightening, as it really is.

We, as members of today's society, need to learn more about depression to change old-fashioned and closed-minded attitudes and progress to the supportive healing process. Clinical depression has become almost epidemic in its prevalence. We dare not dismiss this illness as something trivial and self-indulgent, denying its existence because of lack of knowledge. The lowest form of nastiness is refuting (through sheer ignorance) an illness that clearly ruins so many lives.

The purpose of this book is to inform the reader about the link between dieting and depression; to remove the stigma of depression and to find ways to make the treatment of depression foolproof and specific. But until then, depression can only get better if we abandon our old-wives' ideas of the disease, and start afresh with humility, empathy and an inquiring mind. And most of all, a desire to do good, and help others in need – not kick them when they are down.

Just because depression isn't visible, doesn't mean that it is not a very real disorder. And just because we know so little about it, doesn't mean that we have no means of treating it. And just because it is in the brain, does not mean that there is automatically something wrong with our minds. In this condition, our thinking is often perfectly normal, it just feels like we 'may be losing our marbles' because the chemicals governing our thoughts are disordered.

DR DORA: The mind-body duality

Are the mind and body separate or are they one? It may sound like a simple question, but it has been plaguing thinkers for centuries. The Eastern philosophers always viewed the healing of body, mind and soul as one task. Descartes, the 17th century French philosopher, drew a distinction between mind and body. He wished to separate what humans do into *voluntary* and *involuntary* actions. Functions like breathing, digesting and heart beat he termed *involuntary*. The body controlled these; and they were studied by scientists. Physiology and anatomy became the fundamentals of medical science. Medicine did not involve itself with the study of the mind, spirit or soul.

Anything requiring *willpower* was considered *voluntary*; and hence involved the mind. Descartes felt that the mind had a relationship to the soul, although it was difficult to understand and was not accessible to science. This distinction was later called Cartesian dualism. It dominated the way the mind was viewed for centuries. Believe it or not, there were many benefits to this distinction. For one, early anatomists were given permission to dissect cadavers because they were now considered simply 'dead bodies' without a soul or mind. So the study of medicine advanced greatly in certain fields.

But centuries later, philosophers became uncomfortable with the split between mind and body. Scientists also began dissecting human brains, trying to map out which parts were responsible for which actions. It now transpires that the mind controls the body and the body controls the mind. Understanding the brain as a *physical organ* has helped bridge the gap between mind and body. Exactly what happens when we think, dream, express ourselves and experience the world can be understood in terms of nerve cell function. We have moved far beyond Cartesian dualism, as you will learn.

As with the story about the paraplegic above, people do not ask if it is uncomfortable or difficult to live with the affliction of paraplegia. They just know that it must be. They don't say things like, 'But you still have legs, just like mine! If you train them hard enough, they'll work just fine again! I've had lazy legs, before, and this is how I got them strong again!' I mean, if you heard this being said to a paraplegic, wouldn't you immediately jump in and tell that idiot how completely ludicrous they were being! Wouldn't you automatically want to sit down with that moron and tell him how paraplegia 'worked' to prevent him from ever making such rash and ludicrous statements again?

I think you would. And that is why I am writing this book: to tell you what a similarly difficult affliction clinical depression is, and how not to allow people to get very sick and possibly die because of ignorant, self-righteous ideas.

So, let's move onward and upward, towards the understanding of depression, and start giving more, healing more and helping prevent depressive intolerance in our society.

2 WHAT IS STRESS?

Stress has become a very trendy word. It is an all-embracing condition sweepingly used to explain away all our ills and 'weaknesses', but its broad dictionary definition casts a revealing and useful light on the concept. The **Oxford Dictionary** begins its definition of stress as follows:

Stress/n.&v. a demand on physical or mental energy.

Stress in fact means putting any type of pressure onto something. Carefully considered, it can be a very good thing. For instance: You have an operation and are required to remain in bed for two weeks. During this time your muscles weaken and your fitness level obviously decreases. Then, when your body is recovered, you get back to your daily walk, and now find it quite tricky. You run out of breath easily, and feel very weak – as if your threshold for fitness has increased.

So what do you do? Do you simply stay at this new level of unfitness because you've been weakened by a long convalescence? Of course not! You adapt your training programme to improve your fitness by pushing your muscles, heart and lungs a little more than is merely comfortable. You will also find that your body likes it. It is beautifully equipped to deal with this increased expectation of functioning and it responds positively by improving its output a little more each time. Our bodies apparently like being pushed to 'blow away the cobwebs', as it were.

This is a stress. And this stress is good. Stress on something is positive, as it usually means an upward shift towards improvement and productivity. But, just as with anything at all, too much of a good thing is no longer positive. And as humans we can't resist the temptation to push everything to its limit, with a presumption of invincibility that is humbled only by complete catastrophic collapse!

DR DORA: Stress: good or bad?

We all 'know' that excessive stress is bad; but who would deny that the adrenaline rush of a deadline is a great motivator? So is stress always negative?

Working in the first part of the 20th century, Hans Selye was the first to define how humans respond to stress. He proposed that we first experience stress intellectually; then our bodies adapt to the situation in an *automatic* way through stress hormones such as cortisone. Selye called this response the general-adaptation syndrome. Initially, mild stress can be a good thing; it increases creativity and encourages productivity. The body quickly adapts to the new situation and survives. It is only when the challenge of stress becomes overwhelming or prolonged that the body cannot cope.

But what exactly is stress? It has always been difficult to define or measure, even though we constantly refer to it. Stress is the interaction between the demands of a situation and an individual's ability to cope.[1] Holmes and Rahe were the two researchers who made a breakthrough when they identified that *change* produces stress. Change disrupts the flow of life. Change is stressful, even if it is something we have looked forward to for months – such as moving home, a new school, promotion at work, or marriage. Holmes and Rahe questioned hundreds of people and devised a scale of life changes they called the social readjustment rating scale.[2] The higher one's score on this scale, the higher the likelihood of developing illness later on. Death of a spouse scores a maximum of 100 points. Major change in eating patterns is stressful, quite apart from affecting neurotransmitters and nutritional status, and scores 15. Getting a traffic ticket is considered minor: it gets the minimum score of 11 on the scale! A total score of 200 or more in a single year greatly increases the chances of getting physically or mentally ill.

Research has repeatedly proven that stress contributes to the development of both psychiatric and physical illness. So, change causes stress; excessive stress in one year causes illness. What about ongoing, relentless stress? When animals are subjected (in rather cruel studies) to chronic, unpredictable stress, they become irritable and restless. Giving rats electric shocks, irregular meals and interrupting their sleep causes them to stop exploring their environment. This behaviour is reversed by giving them antidepressants.

It is not simply the chronicity of stress that affects us. The way one views the stress is also crucial. A pessimistic view of stress will definitely make it harder to endure. If the stress is unwanted and unexpected, one struggles to adjust. Trying to find some *meaning* in the challenging situation helps. Many psychotherapies will 'reframe' stress so that something enriching can be extracted from it.

More and more evidence is emerging about the link between mind and immunity. The cells of the immune system (monocytes) are undoubtedly affected by stress hormones and adrenaline. If animals are placed in a stressful situation from which there is no escape, their white blood cells drop in number and they do not produce antibodies.[3] This means that they cannot fight off infection. Studies in humans have also confirmed that under stress, people are more prone to infection and cancer. For example, people who are unemployed, are writing final exams, have recently been bereaved, are caring for parents with Alzheimer's dementia, getting divorced, or elderly people who are neglected all have compromised immunity.[4]

A warning: stress and illness are not connected in a simple cause-effect relationship. The thinking in psychiatry now proposes the 'stress diathesis' model. This means that all people have an underlying vulnerability (diathesis) to illness; and the amount of stress they are exposed to will determine whether or not they get sick. Take epilepsy, for example. For some people, the threshold to developing epilepsy is very low. Let them have a high fever in childhood and they will have a fit. For other people, it takes much more stress to produce a fit. If 10 people are placed in a room with flashing strobe lights, one person might have a fit after five minutes, another after an hour, another not at all. So it is a combination of the underlying vulnerability and the amount of stress that produces illness.

We all test the outcome of the extremes of the stress we place on ourselves, oblivious to the consequences, as if our god-like status in the world somehow guaranteed us against failure. We successfully deafen ourselves to the physical messages screaming from our bodies, and shrug them off as human weaknesses (something, of course, none of us wants to admit to having!) We have realised the power of our brains and now we have pushed ourselves to our physical limits.

Stress that occurs too often, or over too long a period of time, poses a huge threat to our health – and to life itself. In fact, stress plays a causative role in over half of all human disease and death! The World Health Organisation concluded from extensive studies that there are 10 major causes of death, which account for approximately 80% of all known deaths in the First World. Stress is implicated in nine of the 10 (these being heart disease, suicide, strokes, injuries, homicide, cancer, liver disease, emphysema and bronchitis). The most common presenting disorders are anxiety and depression.

Growing up

As children grow they discover new potential with each new stage and test its limits until they are ready to move on to the next level. A newborn baby requires immediate self-gratification and is wholly dependent on basic functions: eating, sleeping, growing and staying alive. This hedonistic set of needs is spawned by what Freud calls the 'id'.

A year or two later, the toddler realises that not only can she walk, but she also has two powerful and creative appendages: hands. She starts touching, feeling, becoming aware; explores the world around her and starts increasing her own sense of control over her environment and herself. Simple routine becomes important, and comfort is derived from repetition and power in self-control.

Her development moves forward to Freud's concept of the 'ego', which gives the child her first conscious control over what she does within her environment. She no longer merely gives in to the primary needs to eat, sleep and drink; she awakens to being able to control her physical needs until they are appropriate.

This is a powerful realisation, and she starts taking full advantage of this independent thought. Until she pushes it too far. She may start wanting things done her way, as the autonomy is a good feeling, and then she will continue, until she realises that too much of this actually causes problems within her environment; it conflicts with the interests and needs of others, and the forces of nature and society conform her to a moderate state of control and giving. This is a major learning curve for her self-worth, and provides her with the foundations of mutual respect and humility.

At an age of between five and 10 she realises the next stage of Freudian development, towards the influence of the 'superego'. This takes the level of control one step further, discovering the higher power of the brain: the independent ability to reason right from wrong and develop a personal opinion of higher-level issues, such as spirituality, religion, a higher awareness of one's surroundings, and of those issues that are not directly related to the individual's well-being.

So, the developing little girl starts acting out this superego, and explores empathy, questioning issues and generally developing her own opinions and values in her future life. This makes her feel more secure, and she is at a very stable level of development.

The next step moves her into a period of chaos as she enters puberty, and suddenly her finely mastered body begins barking back instructions at her. She develops adult physical features, she starts a sexual cycle (whether she likes it or not!) and her mental functioning seems to start the cycle all over again. She discovers new issues that challenge her as a new, young adult, and her self-confidence dwindles in the face of uncertainty. (This throws one a little, but I believe it is all in the cycle of renewal and positive stress. Without it, we would not move forward, onward and upward!)

So, she begins to discover parts of her body she did not know existed, she finds new hedonistic needs arising that resist control as powerfully as hunger and sleep, and she now has to master these as well. In other words, just when she thought it was safe to start living, along came a whole new metamorphosis to throw her confidence completely. You can see why adolescence is such a tumultuous time!

DR DORA: Development of humans over time – Freud's theory

Developmental theory is a branch of psychology that examines how humans change over time. At each stage of the life span, emotional and intellectual functioning, as well as relationships and behaviour are examined. Developmental theories put forwards reasons as to why we behave in certain ways at certain times, taking into account genetic factors ('nature') as well as environmental factors ('nurture'). This has given rise to the nature-nurture debate, when theorists argue amongst themselves about what causes illness: bad genes or bad environment.

Sigmund Freud was the founder of a movement called psychoanalysis. His theories about development have been very influential in fields ranging from psychiatry and the social sciences to art, politics and literature. Until he was in his seventies, Freud continued to develop and modify his theory of development. The theory is immensely complicated and will be sketched in only the briefest outline here. Two important claims lie at the basis of his theory:

- The first few years of life are the most important in shaping the personality.
- Human sexual development begins at birth.

In the early part of the 20th century, when he developed his theories, these ideas were revolutionary.

Freud identified four distinct developmental stages as well as a period of latency (where not much happens). Each stage was named after a different body part, which Freud thought to be the focus of sexual excitement at that particular time. Each stage follows in the same order in every person. The stages build upon each other, layer over layer, and do not replace what has come before.

▪ The oral stage

From birth to a year, Freud termed the oral stage of development. During this time, the baby experiences the world through its mouth. Sensation that derives from the mouth is often pleasurable. In fact, Freud considered it the first 'sexual' experience. In addition to pleasure, the infant may also experiences *frustration* if food is not available. Freud also believed that *anxiety* is felt from birth. During the oral stage, the infant attaches to the mother with the first and strongest love relationship of its life. By the end of the oral stage, the infant has the beginnings of a personality.

Freud believed that tiny infants have strong desires and urges that he called *drives*. In the baby, these urges are largely physical (hunger, thirst, touch) and they need immediate gratification. The structure containing these primitive drives Freud termed the *id*. Screaming for what you want and wanting it *now* works for infants, not adults. As development progresses, Freud believed other channels appeared for our needs to be expressed. He called these the ego and the superego.

▪ The anal stage

Freud named the development that occurs between one to three years the anal stage. During these years, the toddler interacts more and more with the outside world.

Through toilet training, she learns how to control her bowel sphincter. Freud believed that this was the first experience of self control as well as the first contact with the authority of the adult world.

During this stage, the toddler starts developing an *ego*. The ego interacts with the world in a less demanding way than the id. The child starts to learn how to delay gratification and to use logic, problem solving and memory in order to get her way. The urge comes from the id, and the ego decides on how to achieve the goal. Freud compared the relationship between ego and id to rider and horse. The horse (id) provides the energy and power to get to a place; but the rider (ego) guides the animal and chooses the best route.

■ The phallic stage

Between the ages of three and five years, children begin to explore their genital area. Freud believed that children of these ages become possessive of their parent's love. This stage is called the Oedipus complex and is different in boys and girls.

■ Latency

From the age of five to the beginning of puberty, there is a period of calm where there is no new form of sexual excitement. By the time the child has reached latency, the physical drives are not as urgent as earlier in development. The *superego* develops during latency. The superego is similar to a conscience, which tells the child what is right and wrong. It also sets standards of behaviour. The ego is like the parents: monitoring, demanding, rewarding and punishing behaviour.

■ The genital stage

Once the child reaches puberty, Freud believed in a re-awakening of the sexual urges that were dormant during latency. Sexual impulses are (usually) directed towards the opposite sex. Romantic love develops. By the end of adolescence (the genital stage), the ego is pretty stable and it is possible to deal with the demands of the adult world. Freud thought that adults needed to establish a balance between loving relationships and work.

Unfortunately, we adults often forget how difficult a time adolescence was for us too, and the adolescent gets a double-whammy of self-doubt: she thought that she had it all made, and that she had successfully mastered the complexities of life, and then in adolescence she is smartly proved wrong! Now you, as the parent, lose your patience and temper with someone whom you, too, thought had grown up enough. The adolescent really does not like what this appears to be: 'proof' that her development may not have been altogether successful, and that she is being punished for having what appears to be 'naive' self-pride. She thought she had mastered her own body and its place in the environment; meanwhile her underlying insecurities are exposed. She is not in control after all!

Now, I believe this can pose an enormous problem for the child whose development up to this stage has for some reason been hindered. Her development through the physical, to the mental, to the emotional and spiritual may have been interrupted or slowed for reasons of environmental trauma.

Let's take a look at Maslow's notion of development. According to Maslow, there is a hierarchy of development, from the survival mechanisms of eating, sleeping, self-defence and self-preservation, right to the top of the hierarchy towards self-actualisation and advanced decision-making. He hypothesised that we, as humans, cannot progress 'up' to each of the new levels of personal development, until we have fully realised and satisfied the previous level.

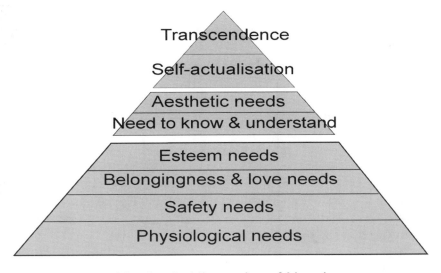

Maslow's Hierarchy of Needs

Street children often run away from abusive homes where they have been neglected. They choose to live on the streets, fending for themselves, with each day being a struggle to survive. As at home, these children live without parental care or supervision. As a result of this lack of care, the child is precluded from developing further than the survival stage, because his survival is always at risk. This child will have difficulty in completing or even attaining any level above that of mere survival. This means that the child's ability to function 'appropriately' in a more advanced society is hindered. By this, I mean that when he is hungry, he will not wait until it is supper-time to eat. His basic drives are still in control, subconsciously telling him that if he doesn't eat now, he may not get a meal. So, his behaviour may change to allow him to eat, even if this behaviour is rough, rude or inappropriate in society. It is obvious, therefore, that because he has not been able to master the next level above mere survival, conscious opinion about right and wrong is almost a ridiculous expectation, let alone a successful feat.

Moving one or two steps further in child-care and development according to Maslow, the child may not have her survival threatened by lack of food, safety or shelter, but her development beyond appropriate physical control may be hindered. She may be struggling to control issues of appropriate behaviour because she was never encouraged and praised in her home environment. Her parents may project their own feelings of inadequacy or shame onto the child, and so she never feels that her efforts to perform appropriately in society are successful or acceptable. Her energy is constantly employed in the futile effort to attain social acceptance within her family, which she never receives, and she is prevented from adequately developing advanced decision-making skills and a higher level of consciousness.

Thus, by the time other children are exploring the higher function abilities of decision-making, empathy, spirituality, higher awareness and advanced, non-selfish thought, this child is still searching for appropriate and acceptable behaviour. This, in itself, instils further feelings of inadequacy in the child, and so lack of development can become pathological, or 'problem-causing'.

The child then enters puberty, and is introduced into the physical world of adulthood. This stage is filled with urges that are as powerful as those experienced in early childhood, and yet there is a conflict; before, the child simply had to control physical feelings until it was appropriate, by which stage the 'wait' was rewarded by, for instance, a full and satisfying meal. Now, a new urge is not only there, but is deemed completely unacceptable to the point of taboo, and is shamed if it is there at all!

What's more, many of these physical functions can be completely unavoidable or uncontrollable, no matter how unacceptable they are. For instance, for a girl, the menstrual cycle is not only kept secretive and shameful, but it is also often seen as an embarrassing part of a young girl; an overt sign of sexuality at an inappropriate age, according to society.

This may be an unfortunate cultural view, but the child who has moved through development in a stable and caring environment usually copes well. In the child who has not been able to move beyond a certain level, however, I believe that this may be where part of the problem lies. The adolescent is overwhelmed by these new changes, when the previous issues have not yet been explored and mastered effectively. So, a bottleneck of developmental pressure ensues, with the child believing one of two things:

- That he/she is not as 'clever' or as 'good' as other children; a deep-seated frame of mind that I believe lasts a long time, or
- that he/she simply cannot cope at all, in which case a breakdown may occur. (By a breakdown I mean the child initiates a pathological behaviour pattern indicative of affirmation-seeking, or complete apathy towards trying to cope.)

This, I believe, may be a reason for eating disorder initiation, as an attempt to assert one's control over one's body (especially if the environment is not conducive to 'smooth' development) and to prove beyond reasonable doubt that one's success is unquestionable.

I will examine this in greater detail later, but by this stage the adolescent may have so little faith in her own abilities to control her environment and herself, that she seeks to gain acceptance from outside sources in an extreme manner. This way, she is reassured that there is absolutely no room at all for doubt in her ability to control herself, and thus reach the socially appropriate level of development among her peers.

Moving back to this model, psychologists generally agree that humans progress and evolve through a series of developmental stages. During this time, several stages of uncertainty are encountered (one being puberty), often 'unsettling' the person's confidence in his or her developmental success. When this happens, such a cycle is re-entered in order to complete it successfully. If the first 'cycle' is completed with relative success and social approbation, then the cycles thereafter will be easier to cope with, I believe. 'Smooth' development, though, is well-nigh impossible. If it were all smooth, there would be no need to develop. Why develop or change if there is no need?

DR DORA: How identity develops – Erikson's contribution

Erikson was a follower of Freud who left Vienna to live in America. He was trained in the Montessori method of education and was also a psychoanalyst. After he spent some time studying Native Americans, he became particularly interested in how humans relate to society. He believed that we develop a sense of social responsibility just as we develop the ability to think and communicate. In order to do this, we need to develop our own identity. Erikson's contribution was that he added a *social* element to Freud's theory of development. To each one of Freud's stages of development, he correlated a 'psychosocial' stage. He described the 'eight stages of man'; where each stage is characterised by a particular struggle that needs to be resolved before we can move on.

Erikson divided childhood into four stages. He believed that in the first stage, there was a battle between *trust and mistrust*. From birth to a year, Erikson believed that the infant must learn to count solely on her mother for feeding and comfort. Ultimately, the baby learns to trust herself, from having had the experience of a caring mother. She can then develop confidence in the world. Mothers must also have faith in themselves as parents during this time. From one to three years, in a stage corresponding to Freud's anal stage, the toddler struggles between *autonomy and shame*. At this time, the toddler is becoming independent. As she begins to walk, feed herself and talk, she learns more about the world. Of course, she still needs her parents' care, and cannot completely achieve autonomy. When her parents leave her somewhere, she suffers from anxiety. When she fails at something and they reprimand her, she feels ashamed. At this stage, there is conflict between the toddler trying to master her environment and her parents wishing to control her. Heard of the 'terrible twos'? This is the reason for the struggle and tantrums. The three to five year old begins to explore the environment in a creative way. Children mimic adults (notably their parents) at this time. They play doctor-doctor or housie-housie. Erikson termed this stage *initiative versus guilt*. The child is either very adventurous or terribly guilty about 'naughty' goals, such as being aggressive or fighting. The last stage of childhood occurs during the equivalent of Freud's latency. The child vacillates between *industry and inferiority*. Erikson believed that now, children become busy and skilled in the world of school. They operate more and more within their peer group. If they fail, they feel judged and inferior.

Adolescence is a time of forging an *identity versus having an unclear role* in the world. Adolescents explore new ideas and new experiences; they hero worship. Thinking about the future, they experiment with different possibilities and roles. They also experience sexual urges and they are dependent on their social group for approval.

Describing early adulthood, Erikson drew on Freud, who emphasised the goals 'to love and to work'. Adults seek *intimacy versus isolation*. Later on, during middle age, the tasks are *generativity versus stagnation*. Erikson believed that at this point, adults needed to raise their children and establish their livelihoods. These adults have a sense of faith in the future. Finally, in old age, if one has achieved a sense of satisfaction from a productive life, one feels *integrated*. If these goals have not been met, the result is *despair* with a fear of impending death.

From this, it is evident that stress can be extremely beneficial when nudging a person along to progress through life. However, when circumstance causes an unnecessary bottleneck of unfinished development, this stress becomes too much to bear, like a dam wall breaking. This induces varying degrees of destructive, anti-social and pathological behaviour that is extremely difficult to correct.

This leads us to the second definition of stress according to the **Oxford Dictionary**:

Stress/ n.&v. strain, burden, anxiety, worry, distress, pain, grief, suffering, anguish … **resulting from continuous stress.**

Here, something that is necessary and good becomes excessive and harmful. It is the transition from moderation and temperance to excess and danger – that is, when good stress becomes bad and harmful stress.

Think of blowing up a balloon. In the initial stages of blowing air into the rubber, there is so little stress on the material that it does not take appropriate shape, colour or turgidity to make it pleasing to the eye. Then, as the air pressure increases, so the stress on the rubber increases and the balloon takes the appropriate level of colour, form and shape. If the balloon is inflated even further, the stress on the material becomes too great and begins to cause damage.

What signs do you receive that this is occurring? The colour becomes too pale, there is a faint sound of strain, the back-pressure on your lips becomes too great, and you really have to pucker and blow very hard in order to maintain this pressure! What's more, there is a strange silence – the 'calm before the storm' – just before the inevitable BANG! The balloon bursts! The material has now 'fatigued' and the excessive stress has forced the balloon to return to its original, flaccid state of zero stress.

This state has been achieved via the most direct route in opposition to the stress, namely destruction to zero stress. The entire balloon was destroyed because the back-pressure warning signs were not heeded. If they had been, then it would have been able to return to its optimum stress level, and stayed there for a long time, giving maximum productivity and pleasure!

I hope, by now, you have followed the inevitable analogy! Humans are like balloons: when we are flaccid or unused, we feel useless and worthless. We cannot contribute in a way that proves that we have a valuable and acceptable place in society. Thus, too little stress is a negative stress in itself!

If, however, the stress is too much, there will always be clear warning signs. If these are not heeded, then nature strikes back in an angry, violent and destructive manner – with disease. And here we have the subject matter of this book: how stress, whether environmental or derived from a physical aberration, can result in disease – disease of the body as well as the brain. A disease called depression.

How stress works in our bodies

We have a complex 'cascade' of hormonal and neural reactions to stress, together known as the 'fight-or-flight' response. This is the body's ability to gear itself up, extremely rapidly, to be able to defend itself from harm, or to seek out satisfaction for a mounting stressor (for example, the drive felt by a lion chasing after a buck when the stress of hunger builds up).

So, this reaction is largely based on the effects of a substance, or factor, called adrenaline (otherwise known as epinephrine). When needed, adrenaline is rapidly released into the bloodstream and transported with immaculate efficiency throughout the body, priming every part, perfectly, to cope with the stressor rapidly and effectively. This magnificent phenomenon continues right up to the moment that the stressor is completely removed. At this stage, there is no further need for this stress reaction, and the adrenaline production stops. Makes wonderful sense, doesn't it?

Take, for instance, your life as a caveman or woman. You stroll out of your cave, and whilst humming softly to yourself and picking juicy, ripe berries, you hear the roar of a lion nearby. What happens to your body at that moment perfectly describes the adrenaline-driven response: your immediate instinct (and that is what it is, rather than a step-by-step conscious thought process, which takes too much time) is to act – fast! Your pupils dilate to take in everything possible, your pulse rises, to deliver blood to all parts of your body that are needed for rapid physical activity. Your blood also moves away from your stomach and internal organs, and towards the legs, arms and heart to deliver nutrients and oxygen to where they are needed. Your breathing automatically becomes more rapid, to fill your blood with oxygen ready for the activity. Your mouth dries up, as you are in no state to start eating! And your muscles all become taut and ready to jump, thrust, hit, kick or run – very fast! You begin sweating in anticipation of an increased body temperature in exertion, and your entire metabolism is rapidly geared to processing energy for immediate use. All this in a split second!

As far as I'm concerned, the body is nothing short of magnificent; an entity capable of transforming from a nibbling, humming and relaxed stroller into an alert and powerful athlete, capable of strength and speed otherwise thought impossible. Incredible!

This stressor is a lion, threatening your life. On a smaller (but equally powerful scale), thirst signals a similar threat to your life: dehydration. When you get thirsty, a mild stressor tells you that you need water. If you ignore this warning long enough, the stressor increases its signal by inducing a fight-or-flight response (your search for water becomes more acute, and consumes much of your thought process). If this is still unheeded (through drought, for instance), the fight-or-flight response will kick in with an aggressive drive to find water, regardless of what may stand in the way.

When the stressor is further disregarded, it will build up to the point of causing a complete breakdown: you will cease to search for water and collapse with physical exhaustion. You will no longer feel thirst; your body will progress beyond the feeling. A process of self-protection starts, as you experience mild euphoria, but with this there will be ensuing physical damage such as kidney failure and death is inevitable.

If however the signal is acted upon (you find water and drink some), then the stressor will decrease incrementally. If your thirst is desperate, but you only satisfy some of it by a small amount of water, then clearly the stress response will decrease, but by no means stop! In fact, the thirst stressor is now so great that in order to 'use up' that fight-or-flight drive, enormous amounts of energy are directed into ensuring that the stressor is 'expended' or satisfied completely. If you provide only half the relief; it will only relieve you of half the stressor! There is still the rest of the fight-or-flight response that has not been satisfied or relieved. It will only stop the stressor response once you have given it sufficient water to relieve the stressor. Not before then – only when it has received what it knows to be enough.

Your system adapts much faster to relieve a stressor than we give it credit for! In fact, the body's regulatory mechanism is so fine-tuned that without this system of control, humans would not have survived as long as they have. Your body drives you to eat, drink or sleep. When the need is satisfied by the required activity, it will cease to exist.

I can hear you thinking: If this is so, why do I have a problem with eating? If my body needs a little chocolate, why, then, do I have a problem stopping there? Surely, if this stressor model is true, then why do I get fat? Why can I not give up smoking? Why do I feel like I never have enough sleep?

The answer is simple: Because there is a bigger problem! Something has made you sick! Whether it is a physical infection, an un-'satisfied' life stressor, or just a dieting-induced chemical abnormality causing addiction or disease, you have ended up with a malfunction in a part of your body that needs treatment. And that is what this book is all about: learning about why your body's ignored drives are now building up stressor signals so strong that they are making you unwell.

So often in the clinic I see people who are sick – not from stress, but from an excess of stress. They complain of many other symptoms, mostly physical, and have a sense of their bodies being 'out of control'; feeling as if everything has gone awry. This points to a stressor that has built up (for instance, the need for a balanced lifestyle), and has been ignored for some reason or other.

Now the body starts stretching and venting some of the tension in one way (mild infection) – and it is given an antibiotic. It starts venting its stress in another way (eczema), and it is covered with elastoplast. It vents in yet another way (self-medicating with binges), and is called 'gluttony', further increasing the stress of pathological guilt. And then we call people affected in this way 'weak' because they are falling apart!

Well, what do you expect?

DR DORA: How stress contributes to depression

In chapter 3 we will discuss the importance of genetic factors in depression. The fact that they are very important, but not completely responsible, is proved by studying identical twins who have exactly the same genetic make-up. If depression were 100% genetic, the same rates would be seen in identical twins. But the concordance rates vary between 30 and 90% for identical twins. Another fascinating piece of research done with identical twins is to study those who were separated at birth and raised by different sets of adoptive parents. Here, the genetic factor is exactly the same in the twins, but the environment differs. Rates of depression are closer than would be expected by chance in the twins raised in different families. This must mean that environmental factors play a part ... which brings us back to stress. Many studies have confirmed that stress predisposes to the development of a first episode of depression and subsequent episodes.[5-8] Stress changes the brain in a *physical* way. On a visible level, the release of stress hormones causes brain tissue loss. *Both* neurons and the connections between them decrease with stress. On a molecular level, fewer neurotransmitters are produced and released. Memory also becomes impaired with chronic stress. There is less brain tissue in the memory centre (hippocampus) of war veterans suffering from post-traumatic stress disorder than in controls.[9]

Let's place stress in perspective as it affects our daily living. Remember that this fight-or-flight response occurs as a result of many hundreds of thousands of years of fighting and flying, physically! But human beings have thrown themselves into the sedate corporate world too recently for these reactions to evolve further to being less physical in nature. So when a stressor in the workplace arrives, our body still gears itself up for a battle or flight from the danger. This would clearly be a bad career move either way, and so the responses for such physical actions are left 'unemployed', as it were. It is this plethora of active reactors in the body which have to have some cause, even if it is not to run or fight, so it internalises itself to become physical and mental disease.

Let's go over this fight-or-flight response again ... but keep remembering that it is designed for the physical reaction of running or fighting, which is not being used in our modern society, which specialises in staying put.

The body senses, in some way, a stressful situation that holds danger for us (not a predator with gaping jaws as in early times, but perhaps a deadline that appears unattainable). The thoughts of danger then reach the hypothalamus, which translates these thoughts of anxiety into physical reactions. This immediate response is called the alarm phase.

In this stressful situation, you need to be acutely aware of everything that is around you. You certainly have no need at this point for digestion, urination, or repair, and so your body redirects all blood flow away from these momentarily 'unimportant' areas, and towards those that certainly do need attention: the muscles used for activity.

The body is also going to need vast amounts of energy for this action-response, and so energy is made available from breaking down fats and muscle (in fact, anything to yield energy quickly) into the 'super-highway' of the blood, which carries it straight to the muscles used for action. The body also knows that whenever lots of physical activity occurs, its temperature will increase. This will slow it down, so it starts sweating in advance. Thus when the temperature starts increasing, the body is already cooling itself in anticipation!

This acute response means that the body is extremely ready for action to get rid of the stressor (either by fighting it or running away as quickly as possible). However, there you are in the office, and all you can do in the way of appropriate activity is to start tapping your pen pretty quickly against the table. Now, apart from irritating the hell out of your colleagues, this activity is barely enough to fully utilise the energy that this alarm phase makes available, and so while this feeling of stress persists, we simply have to sit it out. We all know how horrible this feels, and it can make us do some pretty strange things, as well.

Ever snapped at a poor innocent colleague for no reason? Ever felt abnormally fidgety? Ever felt very 'on edge'? You will notice that everything you do during this alarm phase is done very quickly – because your muscles know that you have to act fast to overcome the stressor.

OK, so the panic has set in: you have realised that if you don't meet this deadline, the irritating little twit who is vying for your job might actually get it. Your body is in fighting mode, and all your instincts are telling you to enact this aggression and wallop the twit as hard as you can. But, you are the master of control, and so you continue with the coolest exterior you can muster, with a restraint that would make Gandhi look aggressive. But, the pressure is still there. It will be until the deadline arrives. So, you enter the resistance phase.

The resistance phase is the body's response to a stress that cannot be solved by the alarm phase. It is the phase entered into when the stressor lasts longer than an hour or two. You see, there are energy reserves in the body which are always there in case we need sudden energy in the alarm phase. These are called glycogen, and they are converted to sugar incredibly quickly, for the panic situations that we encounter.

For instance, I'm sure you have heard of unbelievable stories like the mother who accidentally reversed her car over her child, jumped out, and lifted the car off the child with her own two hands! Now, this is a typical alarm phase response; incredible muscular strength and power only possible in such extreme panic situations.

Following this alarm phase of rapid energy mobilisation (making energy available to the body parts that needed it), the body's glycogen stores are depleted. The adrenaline told them, 'Do whatever you can to release energy – this is a life-or-death situation!' – and that's just what they did. Adrenaline during the alarm phase is like a mayday signal: it does not think of the future; it simply does everything in its power to save our soul from the here and now – what happens after that can be dealt with if we survive!

So, if the stressor continues, and our mayday signal was not successful in removing the danger, the resistance phase is entered into. Though the glycogen stores are completely depleted, energy demands are still high: adrenaline is still there telling us that we need to continue fighting or fleeing the danger because it still poses a threat to our wellbeing.

Also, it is clear that our nerves are still firing on all cylinders, and this requires plenty of sugar. Nerves can only use sugar for energy, so the blood has to have a decent supply of it, otherwise these active nerves start deteriorating. (Now can you begin to understand how shockingly dangerous it is to try and diet during stressful times?) The stored sugar supplies are exhausted, but the body still needs all this energy. So the manufacturing plant in the body switches on: growth hormone and cortisol are released. Adrenaline is still being produced, but because the stressor is longer in duration than adrenaline could be effective in, the body has to employ these other two hormones, which keep the body in a 'heightened' state for a longer time.

These two hormones travel through the blood and start getting energy from two other sources: the fat in storage as well as the protein from all of our muscles. This is called autocannibalism – literally, when we start 'eating ourselves' for energy because carbohydrates are no longer available. Although it is a fairly drastic measure, it is easy to understand why this process is required, in the light of the circumstances we have created for ourselves!

The broken-down fats and proteins empty into the blood and travel quickly to the liver. Here, this magnificent factory of the body takes the fats and proteins and miraculously turns them into sugar. This sugar then empties out into the blood, and voilà! The sugar level is better again.

Let's recap this: in danger situations, growth hormone and cortisol 'eat away' at fat and muscle, which are delivered to the liver, which turns them into newly made sugar for the nerves. This unbelievable phenomenon is called 'gluconeogenesis' (gluco – sugar; neo – new; genesis – to make). Instead of relying on sugar that we eat, it has the ability to make its own new sugar from bits of our body! But remember that it is not a healthy activity: it is a survival technique signalling extreme measures. Unfortunately our lifestyle has made it seem almost normal, but this is why lifestyle diseases are epidemic today: our bodies are not supposed to behave like this in an ongoing fashion.

Amazing? Yes. Good for us. Not really. But then our bodies have to do something to support us in this crazy, stressful environment we subject ourselves to!

The fats in our bodies are sufficient to last us for weeks or even months of the resistance phase. In fact, this is one of the systems that allow us to remain alive even in weeks of starvation. But just because the body can do it, does it mean that we should force calorie restriction to happen for the sake of getting a promotion or getting thin enough for the forthcoming Barmitzvah? I think not.

The resistance phase cannot continue indefinitely. One of two things will happen: in starvation, the resistance phase collapses with the depletion of fat reserves, and organ failure begins, as the body eats the muscles and organs in our body, for survival. (This includes the heart and all other vital organs). This is how untreated anorexics can die. In prolonged anxiety, hormonal changes eventually lead to the body's demise.

- Cortisol produced for autocannibalism also suppresses the immune system, leaving us utterly open to infection and disease (which will make us more sick than we already are, at this stage)!
- The blood volume is increased to preserve all fluids and electrolytes, and the resultant blood pressure can become dangerously high.
- The body's ability to continue producing these stress hormones may eventually flounder, causing a drop in blood sugar levels and energy availability.

Either way (from hormonal collapse, or starvation), the body enters the exhaustion phase. This is when the body's maintenance measures for survival can no longer cope. The body's electrolyte balance changes, the organs may fail, and energy metabolism is no longer functional.

Holistic medicine

Because each and every change within the body affects every other part of the body, there is a need to move towards a holistic approach to healing. This means looking at the whole system, made up of its respective parts, which all function interdependently. We need to look at the body and find out which part of it 'broke down' first, dealing with the initial stressor and removing or satisfying it. Once that stressor has been dealt with, the rest will naturally get better, unless the ensuing harm has caused permanent damage.

It is senseless to look at the symptoms of the problem only, say an allergy, and remove half of your dietary intake to avoid these symptoms. You need to ascertain why there is a problem in the first place! And to do that, you need to examine the entire body and find out where the problem originated.

In my opinion, some medical doctors only do half their job when they do not attempt to find the baseline cause of a patient's problems. They examine each symptom individually and prescribe accordingly. While the patient faithfully takes all the prescription drugs daily, the root of the problem lies unattended. But something else is happening: too much medicine will also cause stress in your body! An excess of anything will result in disease. Unfortunately all doctors now have to carry the burden of an unsavoury reputation for administering 'a pill for every ill', because of these unscrupulous few who do not treat the patient – only the symptoms.

As a result, these closed-minded practitioners have earned all mainstream medicine a bad name. Because the scales tipped too heavily towards blind, simplistic control by drug therapy, society has attempted to balance the trend by moving in the opposite direction, holding sentiments that no doctors are to be trusted; that drugs kill people rather than the disease; and that anything associated with mainstream medicine must be treated with contempt.

Can you see how we are shooting ourselves in the foot? Just because a few doctors are excessive in their drug-only approach, it doesn't mean that all doctors are like that! Just because excessive administration of drugs causes new problems, it doesn't mean that all drugs make you sick! And just because excessive closed-mindedness means overlooking the causative problem, it doesn't mean that holistic medicine is now solely synonymous with alternative medicine.

I must reiterate what I mean by holistic, because I believe this term has also been misunderstood and misused. Holistic means looking at the following aspects of a person's life, to assess why there may be a causative stress building up and presenting a bit more than just a challenge:

- physical organs (all of them!)
- lifestyle
- exercise pattern
- emotions
- workplace
- household environment
- attitude, etc.
- the brain
- time management
- the mind
- diet
- ambient environment
- spirituality

Remember that the cause of many diseases may be excessive stress. And until we resolve why this stress is there, and find ways of dealing with it, coping with it, or removing it if it is unnecessary, then the symptoms will be noticed physically.

DR DORA: The 'bio-psycho-social' approach

The trend in psychiatry today (indeed, in most medical fields) is to treat the patient as a partner. No longer is the doctor all-knowing and omnipotent. Psychiatrists encourage their patients to collaborate in treatment, to share in the responsibility of improving health wherever possible. The framework for this approach is embodied in the 'bio-psycho-social' model of disease. Here, the *cause* of illness is seen as a combination of factors that work together. Three types of problems cause mental illness and distress. Biological factors – such as infection, epilepsy, brain damage, neurotransmitter imbalance and genetic predisposition – are not the only culprits. In addition, the person's psychological health is critical. One's emotional history and one's personality style both play important roles. For example, depression will have a different expression and a varying impact, depending on the personality of the sufferer. Finally, one's social situation counts too. Support systems, interpersonal contact, family background and poverty are critical in shaping and exacerbating illness. *All* of these areas must be addressed in order to treat an illness effectively. Focusing on one aspect alone while ignoring the others is doomed to failure.

From the point of view of the patient, it is important to be honest, to ask questions and learn as much as possible about the diagnosis. The best outcome occurs when patients take responsibility, are well informed and actively address all the areas that need attention. Remember, knowledge is power!

Please note that I have included physical aspects. This is because we usually 'feel' the symptoms of most stress overload in our bodies as disease. If the overload has caused physical changes in the chemical composition of our bodies and brains, then it can most often be 'helped' back up to health by correct drug therapy. Once the body is better, we are in a better state to reassess why we became ill in the first place, and alleviate the other stressor where it started. If we don't do this, we will simply get sick over and over again, requiring more and more 'drugs', until this in itself becomes a problem.

Sometimes, however, a stressor that is not physical to start with (e.g. the death of a spouse) can manifest itself in physical symptoms, such as sleep disturbances. The sleep disturbance is effectively treated and corrected by taking sleeping tablets for several days, until the stressor has had time to work its way out of the initial trauma, or 'breakdown' phase). As such, short-term drug therapy is very important. It is not used as a means to 'sleep away' the problem. It is simply a very effective method to help a patient cope immediately after a difficult and traumatic episode, and while a multi-disciplinary strategy for coping with the trauma is developed. Once the strategy is in place, the brain's chemicals are able to operate normally again, and the drugs can stop.

On the other hand, trauma like this can have irreversible physical effects. The pancreas, for example, can stop producing insulin after a severe trauma. Trauma is always a dramatic intervention in one's life, and no matter how well an individual recovers from the physiological trauma, the physical damage has often already been done. No matter how well the individual recovers psychologically from the original trauma, this dramatic and irreversible change in the body results in the obvious need for ongoing, lifelong medication, otherwise the person may die. Examples of this are trauma-induced diabetes, stroke or clinical depression.

How do we tell whether the psychological trauma is just that, or whether it has become physical/organic, requiring medication?

By visiting a specialist – either an endocrinologist, a psychiatrist or a psychologist (depending on which part of the body is 'broken'). Often, it requires assessment by many specialists, using their own techniques for diagnosis, to find out where the problem really lies, and then they work together, each treating their 'component' specialities until the patient is stable or even cured.

Once the medical treatment shows results, other preventative measures like alternative medicine can be introduced to strengthen the efficacy of the therapy and ensure its maintenance. Regular aromatherapy massage that provides a 'vent' for the day's stressors is a good way to relax. Acupuncture can be used to alleviate certain symptoms such as pain, while the therapy progresses. Alternative therapies such as these are powerful preventative or prophylactic measures, but cannot be used in isolation for an organic disease. Holistic medicine is effective and powerful, like an orchestra playing in harmony – each component working closely together (not trying to do each other's job) to achieve a dramatic end result in perfect synergy.

Let's return to stress. Stress has become the buzzword for modern humankind as we push ourselves to the limit with a seemingly impervious, resilient body and mind. During the last century, we witnessed the rapid advance of industry and technology, causing a heady obsession with changing anything and everything we want. When our expectations aren't met, the outcome is internalised as a sense of failure measured against our perceived 'bottomless brainpower'. Who the hell do we think we are?

Yes, we have an unbelievable capacity for wisdom, knowledge, technical skill and prediction, but we cannot and will never be able to play God in determining our limits. We cannot be in full control of our bodies – they are finely tuned machines that have been altered to perfection over millions of years. Our brain power is good, but we push it to the point of collapse at our peril! Like a computer that is excessively used, not cleaned, maintained and serviced regularly, body and mind will run inefficiently and break down eventually, if pushed repeatedly to the limits.

We are supposed to work, then rest; stress, then relax; overdo, then underdo; be on the ball, and then get enough sleep to compensate. If we appreciate this ebb-and-flow cycle of energy, just like in any machine, we can utilise the full productivity that our bodies and minds offer. But, if we single-mindedly bulldoze past the 'rules' of nature, something will give. And it is not always a pretty sight.

Warning signs of stress

The initial warning signs of too much stress are plentiful, and provide adequate caution that all is not well before causing the body and mind to give in under the pressure. The stressor is a demand placed on our bodies or our minds, and may also be a traumatic life event. The pattern unfolds as follows:

- demands, stressors or traumatic events
- the stress response (the fight/flight response and initiation of a whole cascade of hormonal changes)
- distress (medical, behavioural or psychological distress).

The symptoms are there, and should be heeded as a sign of too much stress. These include:

- irritability
- sleep disturbances (insomnia and night-wakes)
- mild infection and susceptibility to disease (such as sore throats)
- headaches
- poor concentration, focus and memory
- appetite disturbances
- lethargy and fatigue
- changes in bowel movements (stomach upset, irritable bowel syndrome)
- heart palpitations
- dizziness, light-headedness and lack of efficient focus
- muscle tension and pain.

Unfortunately, the seventies, eighties and especially the nineties brought our potential to a conceited head; we basked in the realisation that we could 'tap into' our full potential, and made it fashionable to ignore the warning signs. When we got flu, we took antibiotics. When the flu reoccurred, we took more antibiotics. With each course of antibiotics, the kickback effect increased and our immunity decreased.

An excess of anything is bad if it happens continuously. So, we discover the power of vitamins. Each time the stressor results in a vitamin deficiency, we merely take more vitamins to make it better and carry on working even harder. As the next problem arises there will be another vitamin to ostensibly make the problem disappear. As we work even harder the problems multiply. Psychotherapy illustrates the need to vent our problems, so we start regular therapy in order to 'cope' with the life we have made for ourselves.

The truth is, this life we have made for ourselves is not necessarily natural at all. We realise that we have the potential to progress rapidly, and yet this stressor is an emotional rather than a physical one, so our natural responses to cope (fight-or-flight) are not appropriate responses. They occur anyway, attempting to gear our bodies up for this stressor, but because it is actually emotional stress, this physical potential is not utilised, but internalised to cause us physical harm. To top this problem, our bodies are not prepared very well to cope with ongoing emotional stress. I mean, we have been physically stressed for millennia, but emotional stress is relatively new to our bodies, and so I believe that emotional breaking point is reached much sooner than the physical breaking point would be.

Being left behind by the Joneses – in whatever form (money, status, appearance, etc.) – appears to be one of our greatest fears; the drive to compete is so strong that we continue regardless. In the process, we become sicker and sicker and instead of fixing the cause of the problem, we mend the breakpoints with plasters. Eventually we collapse (both figuratively and literally). And we still have the arrogance to say that we do not need help! Professionals are there! Not only to help us cope once we have reached emotional collapse, but on a regular basis, to be our 'emotional fight-or-flight' substitute! To teach our minds how to cope with these stressors, so that they don't make us sick!

The more we try to control everything with our minds, the more we are forced to lose touch with our environmental and physical warning signs, and the more nature fights back. Nature works in extremely obvious ways, but our highly advanced brains have lost the most fundamental sense: the sense of self-respect (respecting your body). Respect means listening when spoken to, and answering in a fashion that illustrates this respect. Listening to our bodies is a sense – much like sight or touch – that we tend to ignore to the point of 'deafness', and so our 'sense organ' (the emotion of well-being) is no longer a functioning part of our anatomy.

This is where we have gone wrong. Because we have lost this sense, we are floundering in territory we have not yet learned to master. Just like an individual with a blindfold on, our navigation will have to be by trial and error. We will continuously bash our heads and recover from our injuries until we have developed skills in blind-navigation. Like the blindfolded person, we have chosen to deafen ourselves to our bodies! We insist on continuing with the stressing behaviour, in the blind belief that we have to do this in order to survive. As if there is no other choice.

I believe that there is a choice, and this statement is founded on the body-language we have forgotten. 'When you are lost, follow the rules!' And we have been provided with powerful rules for millennia:

- Listen to body signs of stress and fatigue, which mean: 'Give me a break before you continue.'
- Trust in religion and spirituality. Regardless of the religion, there is always time for recovery: in the Jewish faith, there is the Sabbath, in the Christian, each Sunday should be kept for rest, and so it goes on. The rules are there! Follow them! They work!
- Accept that we are all different and that natural selection keeps a fine balance between different types of individuals. We are trying so hard to be alike (lots of money, the same status, the 'respected' career, and the perfect appearance), that we're becoming like one type of animal, vying for a territory that has run out of space! If there are too many buck in a nature reserve living in the same way, in the same place, and doing the same thing, that territory can simply not sustain the volume of the single species. Natural selection says that the strongest and fittest individuals will survive, while the rest get sick and die. In simpler terms, if we all killed ourselves to become the typical social success stories, lawyers, doctors and architects, then there would be too many of these people! Then, those

that chose the career path because it was 'acceptable' rather than having their hearts in it, would eventually fail dismally. Not because they were not 'good enough', but because their bodies and brains were not designed to do these things, whereas those of some of their colleagues were.

- We naturally do well at things we enjoy, and do appallingly at things we do not; unless we work against ourselves, and nearly kill ourselves to do them. Take me, for example, at The X Clinic. I believe I am a jolly good practitioner, because I am passionate about what I believe to be inside of me, as a vocation. Put me in front of an easel, on the other hand, and the lack of confidence I have with performing in an artistic manner evokes more anxiety than you can imagine! I come from an acutely artistic family, and yet I just don't have it! If I tried to sketch, paint or draw in order to be as good as the rest of them, I would constantly be 'swimming upstream', fighting against the knowledge that this is not what I was meant to be. I mean, the amount of hard work and dedication I would have to put in in order to succeed would be more a feat of damn hard work, than passionate suitability. And how much extra effort that would be! And I am sure that ongoing stress would definitely make me sick – or at least want to die because nothing came easily to me!
- Respect our place within nature and our environment. Every part of the environment is integral to our survival. We must develop our skills within that environment in order to survive, but we cannot attempt to control it and manipulate it with our limited capacity. We are still animals! We are still an a relatively insignificant part of the greater scheme of things! We have an advanced power in our ability to change, predict and adapt, but if we take it too far, as we have been doing, we will fail again! Respect, acceptance and humility are essential binding properties to keep us successfully integrated in our environment. Fight against nature and the natural functioning of our bodies, and nature will always win!
- Honour the old rules of hierarchical respect, not to the point of self-abasement, because this is founded on tyranny or idolisation, but with a healthy humility in the presence of those who are more knowledgeable. This may be through age and wisdom, education and experience, and a healthy respect (rather than fear) of the unknown.

The role of fear

Fear is the little darkroom where we develop our negatives.

In the face of uncertainty, human nature usually retreats to fear. We automatically prepare for the worst-case scenario in order to arm ourselves against any eventuality. This fear usually exacerbates itself 'predicting' all sorts of real and unreal eventualities, and preparing us for the worst of these – just in case.

Now, the human mind does have the capability to imagine the worst, and so the greater the intrinsic fear of uncertainty, the more elaborate the perceived possibilities become. This involves an enormous amount of energy being employed, and 'gathered' (as a mounting and 'ready' fight-or-flight response), to the point of accumulated stress and resultant disease. This need to be prepared for any eventuality depends largely on the extent of fear of the unknown. The extent of this fear and the way it is dealt with often depends on how well the individual has mastered the various developmental stages in life and whether each phase was successfully completed.

If you feel confident that you have the ability to achieve adequate success in a particular field, then you have confidence in your ability to handle future obstacles. This means less fear when you encounter such obstacles. So, the stress response that mounts while you face each new challenge is acceptable and does not result in negative stress or disease.

Once that stress response has been mounted, you will only enjoy relief once the specific stress is directly alleviated. You can practise all sorts of stress-relieving techniques to help 'vent' some of that pent-up energy, but they will not remove the source of that stress, which may be a lack of self-confidence in achieving your own acceptable level of success. Hunt the stress down, listen to it and take immediate action on that signal. It may seem impossible. It may induce fear. However, the fears associated with what you may find are, in themselves, usually unfounded or exaggerated.

For instance, if you become a brain surgeon because you feel it will alleviate your inferiority stressor, you have chosen the profession for the wrong reasons. You may perform just fine; in fact, you may perform exceedingly well. However, you will neither find ultimate fulfilment nor alleviate the mounting inferiority stressor, because money, status and fame cannot 'bandage' your feeling of inferiority.

You will drive yourself to work harder and harder at this job, especially when the stressor is not alleviated. You will believe that increasing physical successes will alleviate the stressor. So, you drive yourself beyond socially acceptable success in order to try and fill the 'hole in your soul'.

In the case above, the feelings of inadequacy may have come from a lack of parental appraisal when it was due, and so the child never fully developed a sense of confidence. This is an intrinsic flaw that no creature comforts or social status can alleviate, no matter how many of them are used.

It is vital to delve into why and how this innate hole in the soul came about, and to fix it, in order to enable a domino effect to occur in a positive direction. If we ignore the drive to fill the hole in the soul and develop increasingly intricate and complex methods to ignore it successfully, the need to satisfy or 'fix' it will simply increase. Nature will not be ignored! And it is to nature, after all, that we owe our very being.

So, let's listen. If the body's messages are ignored, they will only hit back harder, and in a more crippling way. I believe that when we avoid dealing with what is fundamentally wrong, this forms the basis for more and more profound mental and psychiatric disease. We try so hard to cover up our fears and insecurities. We develop so many complex strategies to avoid facing the problem head-on, that the stress built up inside our bodies reaches breaking point and makes us sick. Often irreversibly so.

And this is when psychiatric medication comes in on a therapeutic basis or on a survival basis, necessitating lifelong medication in order to maintain the functioning of something that has been irreparably 'broken'. Like a prosthetic leg. You can't grow a leg back once it has been removed, but you can use an artificial replacement to maintain the original standard of your lifestyle.

This is not the proverbial 'crutch'. It is accepting that you have tried to mend something, but because it has been damaged beyond repair you must either become a martyr to your misfortune, or find a false leg! After all, you are much more use to those around you, sporting a false leg and carrying on with life, than feeling sorry for yourself and pretending that hopping is as effective as walking! If you need a false leg, get one, and carry on with your purpose in life! It's your problem at the end of the day, and no one else should be subjected to your martyrdom when there is an acceptable alternative that will allow you to return to society.

Gosh, how philosophical we have become! Now that we are all deep-thinking individuals, let's return to something more concrete: the physical basis of disease, and becoming more acquainted with our bodies!

What stress does to our bodies

Stress mobilises resources in our bodies to cope with a stressor posing a threat. The nervous system activity is short-lived, but its hormonal effects last much longer, and over a prolonged period of time cause what we know to be distress. This takes the form of a range of medical, psychological and/or behavioural disorders, depending on each individual's particular vulnerabilities. For instance, if your family has passed heart problems down to you genetically, then one of the first manifestations of physical distress from stress would be an increase in blood cholesterol levels, rendering you susceptible to heart disease. Gastrointestinal problems running through your family may mean that your first sign of physical distress will be a spastic colon. Looking at your family history, both physical and mental, will give you an idea of where your genetic vulnerabilities may lie, so that you can watch out for distress manifesting itself to you.

The abovementioned are physical stress signs. How about those that manifest themselves in the brain? Clinical depression is possibly the most common manifestation of distress. Thanks to the advances made in both psychological and pharmacological treatments, it is also one of the most treatable diseases.

Burnout can result from ongoing extreme levels of high stress and striving, resulting in fatigue, lack of energy and emotional exhaustion. People with caregiving roles with little or no support (such as single mothers) are often the biggest group suffering from burnout.

Anxiety disorders affect 16,6% of the population in the United States alone, and anxiety and nervous disability (fatigue at work, exhaustion, infections and headaches, for example) account for approximately 33% of doctor's consultations in the UK. This simply indicates how much of a problem stress is in our society – not something to be glossed over, is it?

Conversion reactions are those where the mind's operational overload affects the body's functioning. Behavioural distress is a sign that a conversion reaction is going on. This means that the mind's operational overload is affecting the body's functioning, resulting in inappropriate attempts to cope with stress and trauma. The following are examples of how this stress can become distress, with effects that are far-reaching, not only to the individual sufferer:

- substance abuse (smoking, alcohol and drugs)
- violent behaviour

- becoming accident-prone when under the influence of stress, anxiety and substance abuse, with recovery time from these incidences increasing with increasing stress
- eating disorders such as overeating, causing obesity and Syndrome X, and undereating, causing immunity problems and osteoporosis.

Distress symptoms are the outcome of an individual's failure to adapt either physically or mentally to a stressor that has become too big for human coping mechanisms. There are different stages to this stress, depending on how many of the warning signs have been ignored. Take note of the following symptoms within each stage, and get a rough indication of the severity of your stress levels. (You may recognise many of these symptoms, and give yourself a fright when you realise how many of them were signals telling you that all is not well!)

First-stage symptoms

Individuals who have taken on a large amount of stress may describe it as being stimulating and invigorating. But the symptoms of distress having developed indicated clearly that the level of stress was beginning to affect mental and behavioural health:

1. Constant irritability with people.
2. Difficulty in decision-making.
3. Loss of sense of humour.
4. Suppressed anger.
5. Difficulty in concentrating.
6. Inability to finish one task before rushing into another.
7. Feeling oneself to be the target of other people's animosity.
8. Feeling unable to cope (whether or not this is verbalised or even consciously recognised).
9. Wanting to cry, or snapping at people at the slightest provocation.
10. Lack of interest in pursuing previously pleasurable activities outside of work.
11. Feeling tired even after an early night, and finding it increasingly difficult to get up in the mornings.
12. Constant lethargy and tiredness.

At this point, the individual is no longer coping with everyday pressures and has crossed the 'pressure-stress' line.

Second-stage symptoms

When the individual ignores the first-stage distress signals, and continues experiencing the stress, minor physical symptoms begin emerging:

1. Lack of appetite.
2. Craving food when under pressure.
3. Frequent indigestion and heartburn, and ulcers.
4. Constipation, diarrhoea or irritable bowel syndrome (spastic colon).
5. Chronic insomnia or waking at 3-4 a.m. and being unable to resume sleep for several hours.
6. Nervous twitches, nail-biting or other repetitive, unconscious actions.
7. Headaches and migraines.
8. Nausea, light-headedness and even fainting. Nausea upon waking is one of the most common emerging symptoms of Stage 2.
9. Impotence or frigidity.
10. Menstrual disorders.
11. Eczema and asthma.
12. Tendency to sweat for no apparent reason.
13. Breathlessness without exertion.

Third-stage symptoms

The worse or more prolonged a stressor is, the fewer and fewer coping mechanisms are left to the individual with which to adjust both physically and mentally. So, the symptoms worsen, and the consequences become more serious. This is where the conversion reaction (turning mental distress into long-term organic and physical distress) becomes a real problem. Unfortunately, this is the time when most people seek professional help, rather than at the beginning of the problem. Manifestations of this stage are grave and chronic diseases:

Generalised depression

Signs of this include:
1. Changes in appetite and weight.
2. Changes in sleep patterns.
3. Restlessness or inactivity.
4. Fatigue and loss of energy.

5. Ongoing feelings of guilt or worthlessness.
6. Difficulty in making decisions or concentrating.
7. Depressed mood or feeling 'down'.
8. Thoughts of death or suicide (sometimes the latter is not mentioned in so many words. A patient once said to me, 'Oh, sometimes I feel that if I didn't wake up one morning – it wouldn't matter.' This comment should be taken very seriously.)

DR DORA: Anxiety is common but missed

It is not at all a rare phenomenon to be mentally ill. Despite the secrecy and stigma around mental disorder, up to 10% of the population suffers from a diagnosable mental illness at any time! Up to half of these mental disorders are anxiety disorders. This makes severe worrying, in all of its guises, the commonest form of psychiatric disability.

Anxiety disorders are common, but often missed by doctors. This is because many doctors are unaware of how lethal they can be. They disregard anxiety as something that can easily be overcome. Just relax, they say. But telling an anxious person to relax is a waste of time. It achieves nothing.

Another problem is that anxiety disorders present to the doctor in camouflage. Few people complain of unbearable worry. Rather, they present with physical symptoms that leave the doctor perplexed.

- They may suffer from digestive tract symptoms such as abdominal cramps, stomachache, excessive wind or frequent diarrhoea. Dry mouth is a frequent complaint. Some people even feel as if they are choking and cannot swallow. The gastroenterologists shake their heads after scopes and Barium swallows have revealed 'nothing wrong'.
- Anxiety patients may present to the respiratory specialist with a feeling of suffocation or panting (hyperventilation). There is no physical cause for the distress.
- Cardiologists are called in to examine 'heart attack' patients who have a perfectly normal electrocardiogram. Others suffer from chest pain, irregular pulse rate and chest pain but the investigations are all normal. These patients are sent home, feeling embarrassed.
- Other anxiety sufferers have predominantly urinary tract complaints or sexual problems. It's all in the head, they are told.
- Neurologists find no cause for the prickling sensations, numbness, blurred vision and forgetfulness of anxiety sufferers.
- Severe headaches, as well as tense neck and shoulders may result in dependence on pain killers and muscle relaxants.

Some patients move away from physical symptoms and present with psychological complaints.

- They worry incessantly, to the point that it interferes with their daily activities. Their worries are difficult to control, which explains how unhelpful it is to say 'relax!'.

- They may always anticipate the worst, living on the brink of potential catastrophe.
- Their sleep may be restless and unrefreshing.
- They may be snappy and irritable.
- Concentration is often impaired resulting in poor work performance or careless errors (which cause even more anxiety).
- They always feel lethargic.

It is important to note that anxiety may be a symptom of another psychiatric disorder. We have seen how commonly it co-exists with depression.

Generalised anxiety

Does this sound like you? A very small job with little significance needs to be done, such as getting your admin up to date. Because the body needs to be quite alert for this task to be completed, adrenaline is released, to get you going and put you on the ball. Serotonin capsules also get released at the same time, in order to 'channel' that adrenaline correctly, so that all your alertness and drive go into that job to get it done sensibly and calmly, but with maximum alertness. If the serotonin nerve is recycling too quickly, however, the serotonin capsules never reach the hypothalamus to do this, and so a tiny, non-threatening job starts registering to the brain that it is actually quite threatening.

DR DORA: The neurotransmitters involved in anxiety

The main neurotransmitter involved in anxiety is called GABA. This neurotransmitter has a calming effect on us. But other neurotransmitter systems are involved too. In fact, they are all interrelated. Affecting one affects the other.

The brain's centre for adrenaline production is hyperactive in some of the anxiety disorders, which explains the keyed up, jittery and on-edge sensations that are so common. Certain receptors for adrenaline are also hypersensitive. This means that even a little adrenaline exerts a powerful response through the receptors.

One of the reasons that GABA cannot exert its calming effect in anxious people is because the GABA receptors are underactive and non-responsive. Medications that increase the transmission of GABA have a relaxing effect on anxious people. Unfortunately, many of the drugs available to act on GABA are addictive. A well known 'drug' that also acts on GABA is alcohol! Newer anti-anxiety medications that are being developed at present will not have this addictive quality.

Serotonin also plays a differing and complex role in the various anxiety disorders. Too much serotonin provokes panic attacks in people who are prone to this disorder. Drugs that cause serotonin to be released, worsen panic attacks.

The person experiencing this situation will commence the job, and then start feeling inappropriately anxious about it, without knowing why. S/he may start rationalising consciously about how this job is just a small one and that it is really not that much of a problem, but regardless of conscious thought, the brain is signalling uncontrolled adrenaline. The mind 'remembers' that the last time this cocktail of chemicals was present, something quite frightening was happening.

So, a process of adjustment takes place. When your accounts don't balance, you go back to the figures and start trying to dig up data which might fill the gap appropriately, as it were. The same happens to the brain. Because it is feeling more anxiety than the situation actually calls for, it starts processing back into its files of thought, trying to find what frightening experience might actually be present, in order for it to rationalise this over-anxious state.

The result is somebody who worries about millions of little, seemingly insignificant problems, which may or may not be present, but are certainly not enough to worry about. But because the brain is already processing this chemically induced response of heightened anxiety, the mind has dredged up all sorts of little stressors which 'justify' the level of stress it is feeling. Remember that to a large extent, our thoughts are a result of the chemical interactions inside the brain. So, to some degree, our perceptions of reality are controlled by brain chemicals, not always the other way around.

The phenomenon described above is otherwise known as generalised anxiety disorder, and is a possible 'cousin' of clinical depression. Surprised? Probably you are, because you are one of the millions of people who thought that clinical depression applied to someone who simply can't stop crying all the time. Wrong! This state of chemical imbalance not only makes us worry about small things, but also has an incredibly wide spectrum of effects throughout the body.

DR DORA: The worriers who worry about everything: generalised anxiety disorder

Do you know anyone who is a constant *worrier*? Does this person display excessive anxiety, with all sorts of physical symptoms? It is possible that s/he is suffering from Generalised Anxiety Disorder.[10] It is a very common condition, affecting up to 8% of the population. It is twice as common in women. Most sufferers say they have been this way for as long as they can remember. Persistent worrying is one of their defining characteristics!

This anxiety disorder tends to be chronic, if not lifelong. Sufferers feel apprehension, worry and anxiety about almost every situation. Controlling the worry is a struggle. Their lives are severely affected by the constant worrying. When the body is in 'adrenergic overdrive', people experience shortness of breath, excessive sweating, heart palpitations, nausea, diarrhoea and 'butterflies' in the stomach. In addition,

- they constantly feel on edge
- they are always tired
- they find it difficult to concentrate or their minds 'go blank'
- they are often irritable
- they complain of many physical problems like muscle tension, shakiness, restlessness, dizziness and headaches
- they cannot fall asleep easily because of racing thoughts or worrying
- frequently, their sleep is disturbed and unrefreshing.

Many areas of the brain have been implicated in this condition and various neurotransmitters are involved. But you guessed – serotonin and adrenaline are at centre stage! This kind of anxiety disorder tends to run in families.

Panic attacks

These are a much more specific form of stress-related persistent anxiety disorder. Panic attacks by definition occur randomly and not in response to a stressful situation. A panic attack is indicated by a period of intense fear or emotional discomfort, in which at least four of the following 13 symptoms[11] develop abruptly and reach a peak within 10 minutes:

- palpitations, pounding heart, or accelerated heart rate
- sweating
- trembling or shaking

- sensations of shortness of breath or smothering
- feelings of choking
- chest pain or discomfort
- nausea or acute abdominal distress
- feeling dizzy, light-headed or faint
- derealisation (feelings of unreality) and depersonalisation (feeling detached or not quite oneself)
- fear of losing control or going crazy
- irrational fear of dying
- paraesthesias (tingling or numbness)
- chills or hot flushes.

These panic attacks can be overwhelming to the sufferer and yet appear 'silly' to the onlooker, who is aware of nothing that can possibly be causing such out-of-place sensations and emotions. The reason for such confusion to both the sufferer and the onlooker is the fact that the sensation is created by chemical changes within the brain (often with little or no stress of any sort being apparent). This chemical change within the brain mirrors the exact response that is 'felt' when an extreme threat is posed to the body. As a result, the brain searches for a tangible cause for this overwhelming anxiety, and this is what causes the sufferer to feel that there is 'impending doom', even if there isn't at all.

DR DORA: Panic disorder is terrifying

The essential feature of a panic attack is a sudden onset of intense and overwhelming fear, accompanied by many of the physical symptoms listed above. During the attack, people with panic disorder genuinely feel that they are going to die, lose control or go crazy. It is *terrifying* to experience the sudden onslaught of these physical symptoms. The obvious conclusion is that the illness is life threatening. The symptoms escalate rapidly and the attack lasts for about 10 minutes. Afterwards, the sufferer may feel shaky and exhausted for up to an hour.

Many people with panic suffer for months or years before reaching a psychiatrist. Over 40% of sufferers never seek help for their panic-related symptoms.[12] Those who do present, land up at the cardiac intensive care unit or the respiratory emergency room. In one study of people arriving at the emergency room complaining of unusual chest pain, 43% had panic attacks.[13] In fact, up to one third of people with chest pain but normal coronary arteries (the blood vessels that feed the heart muscle), may really be suffering from panic.[14] These people are convinced they have an undiagnosed, serious illness. But nothing 'physically wrong' can be found with these people. It is embarrassing to go through the ordeal of a panic attack and then to be told there is 'nothing wrong'. When panic disorder is not recognised, the sufferer cannot make sense of the experience. S/he feels humiliated.

Often, the anxiety that builds up in anticipation of the next panic attack becomes worse than the attack itself. This is called *anticipatory anxiety*. It describes a situation where people are constantly worrying about the next attack. So, even if they have two attacks per month lasting 10 minutes each, the fear of the next attack takes up most of the days in between! This fear can be incapacitating.

Typically, panic attacks tend to occur *out of the blue*. They may even occur during sleep and cause sudden awakening. Unfortunately, sufferers frequently do not understand this. For example, if an attack occurs in a supermarket, panic disordered people will wrongly assume that if they avoid supermarkets, they will be safe from panic. They will not embarrass themselves in public. The thing they fear most after the attack itself, is having a panic attack in a place from which there is no escape. But this thinking is wrong! Panic attacks occur randomly, anywhere. So, the next complication of panic disorder is agoraphobia – a fear of being out in an unfamiliar environment where a panic attack may occur. Many situations are avoided because of fear. These unfortunate people may eventually become completely housebound, unable to drive and terribly lonely.

Panic disorder is three times more common in women than in men. The usual time of onset is during the twenties. Occasionally, it can begin after 45 years or in childhood. When untreated, it tends to be a chronic and debilitating disorder. Panic disorder sufferers are at higher risk for suicide than people suffering from other anxiety disorders. Eventually, they become prone to 'stress-related' illnesses, such as heart disease. Their quality of life is poor. The illness presents with many physical symptoms, so sufferers tend to incur high medical bills. Like many psychiatric disorders, panic disorder tends to run in families.

Treatment for panic disorder ideally includes both medication and psychotherapy. These patients are exquisitely sensitive to side effects of medication, so starting doses must be very low. The school of psychotherapy that has been most effective in panic disorder is called *cognitive behavioural therapy*.[15]

- Here, sufferers are educated about the nature of a panic attack.
- They are taught to interpret their bodily sensations during the attack in a realistic way.
- They are reassured that the attacks can be controlled.
- They also acquire skills to deal with future attacks, such as breathing techniques.
- They are even exposed to situations that occur during a panic attack; but they are taught to master these.[16]

Remember that even though panic disorder is a terrifying illness, it can be treated effectively!

Post-traumatic stress disorder

This is experienced by people who have experienced an extremely traumatic event and who continue to be overcome by its effects.

DR DORA: Re-experiencing horror: post-traumatic stress disorder

The wars, famines, genocides and Holocaust of the 20th century brought in their wake a newly defined anxiety disorder. We hear so much in the media about post-traumatic stress disorder (PTSD). What is it?

PTSD was defined in 1980 in the third edition of the DSM IV.[17] It is a psychiatric illness that occurs in *some people* who have experienced a trauma severe enough to be outside the range of usual human experience. According to the DSM, there are four main components of the diagnosis:

- the trauma is re-experienced
- reminders of the trauma are avoided
- responses are numbed
- sufferers always feel on edge.

In more detail, the *traumatic event* must be severe enough to involve actual or threatened death, serious injury or threat to physical well being, and to cause a response of intense fear, helplessness or horror. Examples of these kind of events include:

- combat experience
- natural catastrophes
- assault
- rape
- highjacking
- serious accidents.

The trauma may be either directly experienced or witnessed. Sometimes, it involves confronting a traumatic event, such as a parent's death. In addition:

- the trauma is *re-experienced* through dreams and even during the day, one may seem to be reliving it
- when one is reminded of the trauma, it causes intense psychological distress, with physical symptoms of anxiety.

Finally, all reminders of the trauma are avoided.

People with PTSD frequently describe themselves as emotionally numb. They are not responsive and they seem detached. Nothing moves them or gives them pleasure. They do not show much emotion. Above all, they have no faith in a lengthy future. As regards their physical symptoms, they are wound up and tense. They are easily startled and they have difficulty in falling or staying asleep. They are prone to outbursts of anger and poor concentration. Sometimes, there is an inability to remember part of the trauma.

The symptoms must persist for at least a month. They must cause significant distress as well as impaired function.

So one might ask: if this diagnosis dates from 1980, is PTSD a symptom of our turbulent times?

It is true that PTSD has been diagnosable as such only since 1980, but it is certainly not a new condition. Throughout history, it has been described and given a number of names. After the Great Fire of London, Samuel Pepys appears to have suffered symptoms. During the American Civil War, 'soldier's heart' caused enormous suffering and disability. During the First World War, it was called 'shell shock'. Many of those who survived the trenches suffered chronic disability. 'Battle fatigue' was the name given to soldiers with PTSD symptoms during the Second World War. Many Holocaust survivors developed PTSD.

But it was the Vietnam War that led to the first systematic study of an abnormal response to major trauma. This was an unpopular, seemingly senseless war in a distant land. Only those with money and connections could escape the draft. The soldiers who returned to America from the war were not celebrated as heroes. Their unpopularity made their suffering worse. Studies of these soldiers revealed that many were suffering from PTSD.[18] Research showed a predictable pattern of symptoms and disability in these people.

There are some parallels to be drawn here with the 'border wars' of the apartheid regime. Soldiers returning from these secret combat situations were also shunned by society. When suffering is meaningless, it is much harder to bear.

How does one make sense of why people develop PTSD?

- Does the extreme stress cause psychological damage? Here one would postulate that the victim is vulnerable and PTSD is a psychiatric illness.

- Is it a normal response to extreme trauma? According to this theory, the perpetrator is responsible and the victim is 'normal'.

The problem here is that most trauma survivors do *not* develop PTSD: it is the exception.[19]

The exact causes of PTSD are complex and multiple. The thinking today is that the *kind of stressor* does play a role in the likelihood of developing PTSD. For example, people who are prisoners of war are at higher risk than survivors of natural disasters. There is definitely an interaction between the event itself, the victim's genetic predisposition, the psychological makeup as well as the environment.

The word 'post' in PTSD implies that it occurs some time after the trauma. The symptoms may start almost immediately or decades after the event. The symptoms wax and wane over time. At times of stress, they may worsen. Frequently, the PTSD does not exist in isolation. Over half of sufferers have at least one other condition such as aggressive outbursts, poor impulse control, depression and drug or alcohol abuse.[20]

There is much that remains to be studied in the treatment of PTSD. Some people feel that early intervention reduces the likelihood of PTSD developing. People who are exposed to trauma should rapidly receive counselling, or 'debriefing'. Others respond that debriefing does not help to prevent the condition from developing. Medication can be used although there is no perfect drug developed as yet for PTSD. Some forms of psychotherapy may be useful in dealing with the symptoms.

All of the above dramatically demonstrates how widespread and severe the effects of stress are, and you may well have felt that I was describing you in some instances. This is why I am writing this book.

Much time is spent in my practice teaching people about the misconceptions regarding anxiety disorders and depression, and the stigma attached to them, before we can get down to the nitty gritty of why they are suffering from lethargy, weight gain or loss, headaches, decreased libido, ongoing infections, chronic fatigue or ME and the many lifestyle disorders associated with Syndrome X such as cholesterol problems, hypertension (high blood pressure), gout and arthritic disease, infertility and ongoing malaise.

So now, when I talk of anxiety, stress and depression, be aware that these terms may, in fact, apply to you - albeit even in a small degree!

Read on and learn where to go.

3 WHAT IS CLINICAL DEPRESSION?

Although I am neither a clinical psychologist nor a psychiatrist, the experience gained in my practice has allowed me to spot when a patient might be suffering from clinical depression. In fact, many people who approach me for help in weight regulation also need help with serious lifestyle and psychiatric problems. If I feel that depression is the underlying problem, I describe the symptoms to the patient. If the symptoms sound familiar, I immediately recommend a clinical psychologist and psychiatrist for professional evaluation and diagnosis.

Just to get the record straight, clinical depression is not only incredibly rife among humans in general, but also tends to be prevalent in women. This is regardless of whether they are rich or poor, employed or unemployed, urban or rural dwellers, and also regardless of ethnic group. It also happens to those women of whom one would possibly least expect it: those who are particularly ambitious and successful. This does not prove that women were not supposed to cope with running a merchant bank, as we shall see!

Many people who are 'adrenaline junkies', 'Type A personalities', 'hyped', 'over-achievers' and so on, are this way because they ride on their overambition and excessive drive to get them where they are today. But what most of them don't realise is that the excessive fight/flight messages that keep them on their toes do so at the cost of physical and mental damage. They are sometimes reluctant to address their problems, because they are afraid that they will lose their drive and not be able to remain successful. Quite the contrary! If their underlying depression is treated successfully, their drive will remain; they will just be able to channel that drive into even more successful productivity, due to controlled physical distress.

What on earth is she talking about, you may be exclaiming. Read on and relax, you uptight thing, you!

DR DORA: Women get depressed more often than men – prejudice or fact?

Depression is primarily an illness of adults. Only about 1% of children get depression. The numbers start climbing in adolescence, when teenage suicide becomes a serious risk. Overall, the majority of depressive people are *adults,* with an average age of 40 at the time of the first episode. It is rare for a first episode of depression to occur in an elderly person, although it certainly does happen.

But depression is not only a disease of adults: it is predominantly a disease of women. All studies of the prevalence rates of what psychiatrists term 'major depressive disorder' show that it is twice as common in women as in men. This finding is always repeated, regardless of who conducted the study, which population was studied and when.[1] Research findings from large population surveys, in many different countries, have consistently shown that women get seriously depressive and anxious twice as often as men do.[2-5] A woman stands a one-in-five risk of getting depression during the course of her lifetime (21,3%). Men have just over a one-in-ten chance of getting depression (12,7%).[6]

Why is this? Is it a true, scientifically substantiated finding, or does it reflect an anti-woman prejudice? The debates in the scientific literature swing backwards and forwards and the answer is complex. There are three main schools of thought explaining the finding. The first attributes the finding to biological reasons. The second blames psychosocial factors for women's depression. The third group discredits the other two and says it is largely bad research methods, prejudice and artefact![7]

Biological factors
We know that women and men have different bodies. But the biological differences go much further than shape and curves.

- The structure of women's brains is different to men's. Women's brains, understandably, have a smaller area sensitive to male hormones. But the tissue connecting the two hemispheres of the brain is much larger in women. In addition, the point of junction that connects the unconscious material from the two hemispheres is *also* larger in women. Emotions are processed in the right side of the brain and language is formulated in the left side. The strong connection between the two hemispheres *in women* means that they can express what they feel more easily. Feelings (such as depression) can be converted into language and given a voice. This means that most women express feelings through words better than men. It also explains why women seem to be more sensitive to other people's feelings than men.

- There are differences in the amounts of chemical messengers (neurotransmitters) released by women and men.

- Women's hormones affect their emotions during the various phases of the reproductive cycle. Hormones play a role in regulating mood.[8]
- Genetic factors are another aspect of biology that cannot be ignored. We know that depression tends to run in families. Genetic material is different in women, who receive the 'x' chromosome. Families therefore pass on different inherited problems to girl children as opposed to boy children.

Social factors
It is not only the structure of the brain that affects how easily women express their emotions and how they deal with stress. Society places different pressures on women and men.

- It is more acceptable for a woman to verbalise feelings of hopelessness than it is for a man. This interaction between emotional expression and socially determined roles is referred to as a 'psychosocial' factor. So from a psychosocial perspective, women are more likely to discuss difficult emotions, such as sadness, than men, because they face less prejudice about being 'emotionally weak'. Perhaps women report the symptoms of depression more readily, which leads to a bias in the statistics and makes it *appear* that depression is commoner in women.
- Women also tend to have more responsibilities than men. They may have several social roles such as taking care of the family, an elderly relative, doing a job and being a wife. This is loading is referred to as 'role strain'. It may explain why women are more stressed than men and therefore more prone to depression. Several recent studies have refuted this role-loading hypothesis.[9]

Artefact
Finally, there may be a degree of artefact in the research.

- The prevalence rates of depression depend on which population of patients is being studied. When we look at those people attending a primary health care centre (a clinic, family doctor or general practitioner), it appears that more women than men are depressed. But we also know that women seek help from a doctor more easily and more often than men! So, perhaps women's depression *seems* to be more common, but actually, clinicians are just picking it up more often.
- In addition, women tend to come into contact with the medical profession more often in their lifetimes than men do.[10] Teenage girls seek family planning advice; pregnant women have regular medical checkups and mothers may see doctors when their children are ill. Depressed women are therefore more easily caught in the net of the medical system.
- Artefact may also derive from the side of the diagnostician. Certain doctors are prejudiced and will easily label women as depressed, but struggle with the concept of a depressed man. Men are more commonly labelled 'alcoholic'. Indeed, research has shown that alcohol abuse is far commoner in men.[11] But we know that many alcoholics have the additional problem of depression. How many men who are dependent on alcohol have an underlying depression?
- Statistics may be biased both by women who readily report their symptoms and by diagnosticians, who label women as depressed more easily then men.

DR DORA: Personality and depression: chicken or egg?

Are certain personality types more prone to depression? Or does depression influence personality development? What is chicken and what is egg?

Several years ago, two cardiologists who were researching blood pressure and cardiac disease came up with a broad classification of personality styles.[12] They called them types A and B. This classification is very useful (even though it was not invented by a psychiatrist!) The cardiologists were studying how certain behaviour patterns may lead to coronary artery disease, which is a major cause of heart attacks. Type A personality refers to driven, ambitious people who are always pressed for time and may be excessively competitive and hostile. Type B refers to the opposite personality style: a relaxed, unhurried, happy-go-lucky sort of person. It was shown that type A behaviour is a risk factor for coronary artery disease.

What about depression? One might expect depression to be more common in the stressed type A personality. But research shows that both type A and type B suffer equally from depression. In fact, depression is equally common in all personality types. However, the difference lies in coping skills. 'Hyped' overachievers will not cope well with the feelings of worthlessness and lack of motivation that so frequently accompany a depressive episode. They cannot tolerate imperfection in themselves. To some extent, the more relaxed type B personality may cope better, but depression is still extremely painful for them to endure.

A very interesting finding in the study of depression and personality is that certain personality features may become exaggerated during a depressive episode. For example, a person who tends to be slightly suspicious at the best of times, may become almost paranoid when depressed. Or a person who is usually mildly obsessive may develop pronounced obsessions when depressed.

It is very difficult to describe what clinical depression is, because the truth is, the medical fraternity is still busy searching for more reasons why it is present in the first place. Let's be quite clear about one thing from the outset: clinical depression does not only mean that you are necessarily depressed. In fact, when I suspect clinical depression and suggest a referral, most patients are extremely offended and react accordingly. 'But I'm not depressed, I couldn't be happier! What have I done to make you think that I am depressed? I don't mope around feeling sorry for myself,' they protest.

DR DORA: How do we define depression?

What is depression? It is essential that the general public understand the *psychiatric* definition of depression because feeling gloomy is so common. Many people have days when they feel 'blue' or are weepy for no reason. When situations become frustrating, fleeting suicidal thoughts may seem to offer a way out. Are these times of feeling low the same thing as clinical depression?

We must also be certain that all doctors mean the same thing when they call a person depressed. In order to standardise diagnosis, treatment and research in depression, some sort of system is necessary. The American Psychiatric Association has formulated diagnostic criteria for several illnesses in a publication now in its fourth edition, called the *Diagnostic and Statistical Manual of Mental Disorders (DSM-IV).*[13] The DSM-IV will be referred to frequently. The criteria for depression include a list of symptoms that must be present in order to make the diagnosis. Depressed mood appears in several different conditions in the DSM-IV, but the one most commonly referred to is called 'major depressive disorder'.

The symptoms of major depression have to last for at least two weeks – but they usually last much longer. We discussed the definition of depression briefly in chapter 1. Let us look at it in more detail. The symptoms of depression can be divided into three clusters:

- mood
- bodily functions
- thinking.

The core cluster is a serious disturbance of mood: feeling low or empty most of the day, almost every day. Depressed people also lose interest in activities that used to give them pleasure. They may abandon their hobbies, and withdraw from friends and family.

The second cluster of symptoms refers to physical rhythms that non-depressed people simply take for granted. Under normal conditions, most people feel hungry every few hours, fall asleep easily when tired, have ample energy during the day and have a sex drive (libido). In major depression, many of these functions become severely disturbed. Depressed people may lose their appetites and slowly lose weight, without dieting. (The opposite can also occur – they self-medicate with 'comfort foods' and gain weight.) They have no energy, may move slowly (or occasionally in a frenzied, agitated way). One of the hallmarks of major depression is disturbed sleep.

Abnormal thinking characterises the third cluster of symptoms in depression. Here, both the way one thinks and the content of one's thoughts are abnormal. Concentration and memory fail. Depressed people are indecisive: even simple decisions seem insurmountable. A negative outlook, excessive guilt and perceiving oneself as worthless, characterises thinking. Recurrent thoughts of death are common. This may even progress to planning a suicide.

The episode of depression causes severe distress and interferes with the ability to function in important areas of life: such as at work, the social setting or in the family. The doctor making a diagnosis of major depression must ensure that the condition is not caused by use of drugs or an underlying medical illness.

DR DORA: The link between depression and sleep

Occasionally, depressed people sleep excessively: perhaps twelve to fourteen hours per day. However, sleep deprivation is much more common. Typically, the nighttime sleep is broken by numerous awakenings. There may be an early morning awakening (at three a.m., for example), where the person tosses, turns and struggles to fall asleep again. Other depressed people find it difficult to fall asleep at their usual bedtime. Depressed people tend to wake up feeling exhausted. They complain that the quality of their sleep is poor. They do not feel refreshed on waking, even if they have slept for eight hours. To understand these abnormalities, it is necessary to explore what the normal person goes through during an ordinary night's sleep.

To begin with, sleep is not one state. Rather, it is a series of four stages, each with typical characteristics. Brain waves slow down during sleep and they can be measured with a special recorder called an electroencephalograph (EEG). When one is awake, brain waves are fast. The deeper one's sleep, the slower and slower the brain waves become. So, in the middle of the day, when one is wide awake, brain waves are rapid. They occur at 8-12 cycles per second (Hertz) and are called alpha waves.

As one settles down at night with a book and becomes drowsy, brain waves begin to slow down.

- **In stage one sleep**, the brain waves become even slower, at 3-7 Hertz. These are called theta waves. Sleep is still light. It is easy to wake a person who has just dropped off to sleep or is in stage one sleep.

- **Stage two** is a slightly deeper sleep, where specific wave patterns show up on the EEG (called sleep spindles and k complexes).

- **Stages three and four** occur when one is deeply asleep. Here the waves have slowed down considerably to 1-2 Hertz (delta waves). If one is woken from stage three or four sleep, one is confused, scared and disoriented.

- **Dreaming** There is a final stage of sleep characterised by rapid brain activity and dreaming. It is called rapid eye movement sleep (REM) because of the jerky movements of the eye muscles that occur. During REM, the skeletal muscles are almost paralysed, and are often responsible for the sensation of not being able to run/walk properly in a dream.

The term 'sleep architecture' refers to the order of the sleep stages, because the four stages occur in a specific order in the normal person. It is helpful to think of the structure of normal sleep like a diamond mine. The surface of the earth represents full consciousness. Stage one sleep is the first level of the mine under the ground. This is a shallow level and the miner can easily be hauled to ground level (full consciousness). Stage two sleep is deeper in the earth; stages three and four are very low down indeed. Getting back to ground level from stage four means one has to go back through stages three, two and one. At this point, REM occurs. The normal time taken to move through the cycles and arrive at the first REM stage is an hour and a half. After this first cycle, the pattern is repeated. During a normal night's sleep, one becomes drowsy, then goes from stage one to stage four, back to stage one and an episode of REM, up to four or five times.

Now that we have outlined what happens during a normal night's sleep, how do we determine what happens when depressed people sleep? The *polysomnograph* monitors the complex changes that the body goes through during sleep by measuring various bodily functions. These include

- brain waves (measured with the EEG)
- eye movements (measured with an electro-oculograph or EOG)
- body temperature
- muscle movements (measured with an electromyography or EMG)
- amount of oxygen in the bloodstream
- chest movements
- airflow through the nose.

When examining the readings from a polysomnograph of a depressed person, several abnormalities become apparent. First of all, in depression, it takes longer to fall asleep. The REM period happens very early and more time is spent in REM. This may explain the vivid dreams that are so distressing. There are numerous awakenings during the night. Patients awake in the early hours of the morning and cannot get back to sleep. Little time is spent in stages three and four (there is little restorative sleep) and most of the sleep time occurs in the shallow slumbering stages one and two. This probably explains why depressed people complain of waking up exhausted.

Abnormal sleep patterns in depression have some bearing on response to treatment, both psychological[14] and pharmacological. Depressed people with severely disturbed sleep tend to do worse with cognitive behavioural therapy than those who are not sleep-deprived.

The responses that I receive from patients when I suggest a diagnosis of depression are both angry and fearful. Angry, because the patient suspects that somehow I have the ability to see into her well-kept secret. Fearful because of the stigma attached to depression and anti-depressants. These responses are usually from people whose minds are their best asset. Often, their perception is that their minds might be tampered with, inhibiting their success; or that they will be forced to take sedatives by the handful, with fading prospects of ever living their lives to the full.

Nothing could be further from the truth! At this point I call for calm – and the opportunity to explain. Simplifying the brain helps to remove the fear associated with its mystery. Please note that in reality this is much more complicated, and here I am calling Mount Everest a molehill – but for a very good reason!

DR DORA: Serotonin does not act alone!

We have already mentioned how serotonin and adrenaline interact with each other and affect each other's release. Many other factors and neurotransmitters are implicated in depression, but they are beyond the scope of this book. Understand that the explanation given here is not completely scientifically accurate. Rather, it has been extremely simplified for the sake of clarity.

Brain-mood interaction

If we are clever, then we are good, by modern standards. If we are clever, we will have money. If we are clever, we will be as good as everyone else. We will be respected. And we will be leaders. We have realised that there is often more power in our brain than in our brawn, and its potential has made us conceited. We control our world through human and artificial intelligence. It is essential that our computer systems and our brains function smoothly – remember the Y2K frenzy? We are now punting women's brains to replace the female body as a symbol of sexuality, just to indicate how important it has become to us.

It is only natural then, that when you are told there is something wrong with that brain – like depression, for instance – that it can be perceived as a major insult.

What makes that 'big, beautiful and sexy brain' so attractive, is that it is individual and human. And the parts that make us human are those that don't always behave 'appropriately': the giggles in a soppy part of a movie; the uncontrolled bursts of laughter during a marital row; or weeping at the sight of a new-born baby. This makes us human; these quirks make us love each other, because they form part of the same, fallible creatures we feel comfortable with. Without the mole, Cindy Crawford simply wouldn't be as nice. The mole makes her accessible, makes her real, the girl next door; not perfect. We feel comfortable with the slight imperfection, because to a certain extent it is perfection that we resent, although perfection is something we conceitedly believe we are all destined to attain.

The little computer-enhanced monster of perfection smiling calmly back at us from the pages of **Cosmo** is viewed as a personal statement of rejection: we've been trying so hard to get there, without any apparent success. We feel as though we are 'not good enough', by comparison. We see the picture, but completely overlook the spray-painted touch-ups, the lighting that takes seven hours to set up, the special filters and million-dollar camera used to create an image of perfection, thinking: 'It looks so easy to get there, but I can't!'

It is at this point that we lose all capacity for logical thought, and forget that this image is not real, but an embodiment of what all of we insecure people have created as our ultimate goal. And because we cannot get there, we feel inadequate, and start looking for other means by which we can appear as successful as this 'Superwoman' image:

- 'Well, at least I'll try and look the part by showing off things that most people associate with mental perfection: a nice car, a nice house and lots of smart clothes.'
- 'You can't get these things if you aren't clever, so this will fool them.'
- 'Even if it kills me, I will have that job/house/car, otherwise who will want me?'
- 'What if they find out that I am not one of the well-rounded, mentally well-adjusted, calm, "together" and "in control" people that deserve a place in society?'
- 'I mean, if anybody happens to notice that I am human, I'll fall into the slippery category of the "untouchables" – unclean, and unworthy of normal respect and public acceptance.'

Sounds melodramatic? Well, then, why do people get so uptight at the mere suggestion that some chemicals may have gotten themselves out of kilter in the brain, as in depression? Think about it. But not too hard, yet. We are still getting to the nitty gritty. And, if you're anything like me, such hard thinking may induce the rather unpleasant odour of burning rubber.

Let's get back to the brain and its functions. The brain has always been seen as the 'mind'; the thought-processing, personalised part of our private beings. This it certainly is, and may also house the spiritual 'soul' as a result. For the moment, however, let's not concern ourselves with that aspect. I simply want to discuss the brain as a functional and structural organ in the body; not our personal perceptions of such functions; merely the biological functions themselves.

The brain has various sections, which are characterised and named by their functions and structure. Deep within the brain, near the centre of the mass, lies a small area called the hypothalamus. This area is well known for being the central 'hub' of information regarding emotional responses.

DR DORA: What is the seat of emotion?

The area of the brain believed to be involved with emotion is called the *limbic system*. It is an unconscious part of the brain, but has many connections to the conscious brain areas. Scientists have known since the 1950s that serotonin is one of the neurotransmitters that regulate emotion because it is found in high levels in the limbic system.[15]

For instance, while watching a horror movie, your visual sensors connect with your conscious sensors. These, in turn, connect with those in your hypothalamus. This processes the thought into a tangible emotion, called fear. The hypothalamus then processes the emotion (fear) one step further: making you feel it physically. This means acting through other parts of the body, such as faster heartbeat, more rapid breathing, widening eyes, and even a mild sweat. All this because of Freddy on the screen!

OK, so the hypothalamus has processed the signal of fear into a hormonal response, by causing the release of adrenaline. This adrenaline circulates around our bodies, causing all the effects mentioned above. But, it also circulates back to the hypothalamus, where it has the effect of registering anxiety in an emotional manner. By this simple little model, one can see how merely watching TV can affect almost every single mechanism in the body. And that is knowing that you're safe, at home, and in no apparent danger.

Moving on, the hypothalamus is the site of many, many functions to do with co-ordinating emotional response. It has a neuroendocrine (neuro – nerve, endocrine – hormonal) function. By this, I mean it is the 'translator' of all nerve messages which arrive from the thinking part of the brain, and turns these messages into hormonal signals, which are then sent out to create their effects. Going back to our movie-watching example, it is the means by which the thought signal of fear turns into the hormone adrenaline, whose effect is to make the heart beat faster. Clever, isn't it?

So, the specialised function of the hypothalamus to turn thought into physical 'feeling' is a very powerful phenomenon indeed, and abuse of this potential is where some problems may arise in us fallible humans.

Let's start by recapping on one reaction, which is both powerful and far-reaching in its activity – the 'fight-or-flight' response, as mentioned in the last chapter. The fight-or-flight response is thus named because it is the mechanism by which our bodies are enabled to deal with those dangers which humans have had to cope with for thousands of years: running away from a dangerous animal; fighting off an intruder trying to steal our food; fighting to protect our young from being taken as a meal for a predator, and so on. It is a very physical reaction, priming us for a very physical response from a very real and physical panic situation.

There are two main messengers or neurochemicals responsible for this response. The brain in fact receives zillions of other messages on a minute-to-minute basis, but here we are concerned with adrenaline and serotonin. These amazing neurotransmitters (messengers) work on the brain constantly to keep our thought processes accurate and appropriate.

Let's start with adrenaline. We all know this one really well in South Africa – it's our 'fight-or-flight' chemical or neurotransmitter. When we are presented with a stressful situation, whether it be physical (someone chasing you!) or emotional (a deadline for work), adrenaline is released, like little balls, and travels through the bloodstream to the brain, where it hits against the brain's surface, eliciting a response of 'alert'. This happens on a small scale, like when we wake up, or on a large scale, like when we literally need to fight or flee, as in a life or death situation (a gun to the head, heaven forbid). As a result, the brain has a way of knowing that alertness is what is needed, whether on a small and gently alert scale, or on a completely huge alert scale!

DR DORA: A psychiatric view of adrenaline

Adrenaline is a neurotransmitter that activates both the body and the mind. Up to 17% of the body's adrenaline is found in the central nervous system. Adrenaline is responsible for the 'revved-up' feeling of alertness. It also assists with learning and memory. It plays a role in the brain's 'pleasure centre' and encourages us to seek rewards. While we are in an alert state, adrenaline helps us focus and concentrate.

Excessive adrenergic activity in certain brain areas is believed to cause anxiety and even panic attacks. In a severely anxious person, the *adrenergic* system is volatile and in overdrive. Brain imaging studies confirm that the adrenergic centre of the brain is hyperactive in anxiety states.[16] Adrenaline plays a role in many other activities, including sleep, appetite and mood.

The low mood seen in depression is caused, in part, by low adrenaline levels. Drugs that deplete the brain of adrenaline cause profound depression. Drugs that increase adrenergic activity lift mood and are antidepressants. Serotonin and adrenaline are first cousins because adrenaline stimulates the production of serotonin. Many of the newer antidepressants treat depression by increasing *both* serotonin and adrenaline levels. Once an adrenergic antidepressant has kicked in, there is more powerful adrenaline activity in the part of the brain that helps with focusing and concentrating. The neurons that produce adrenaline become more active than previously.[17]

Note: In most psychiatric literature, it is referred to as 'nor adrenaline', because this is the way it exists most of the time in the body.

DR DORA: Do the brains of depressives work differently?

Yes they do. There is fascinating research coming out about how the brains of depressed people work. These studies have been made possible because of the new imaging techniques we have available in research. Certain sophisticated brain scanners show us how active or underactive various brain regions are in depressed people, which explains many of the symptoms that are so familiar to the depressive. Amongst other findings:

- Overall, the brains of depressed people are *less active* than normal. *This may explain their feeling of slowness, lethargy and lack of excitement.*

- The brain region controlling *willpower* is also underactive in depression. *This means that it is much harder to get going and small tasks seem like insurmountable obstacles.*

- Those areas that allow us to focus on the outside world and to take in details of the environment are also underactive. *Hence, the depressed brain is more turned inwards on itself.*

- Depressed people lack motivation. *So they seem passive, have no drive or desire to do anything.*

- The area that controls the *meaning* one derives from the world is also sluggish. *So, depressives see no point in continuing. Their lives are meaningless and hopeless.*

On the other hand, certain brain regions are *hyperactive* in depression:

- One hyperactive area is the part of the brain that pulls long forgotten experiences out of the memory, and keeps them in consciousness. *This means that depressed people keep going over old memories of unhappy experiences. Negativity dominates their thinking.*

- Another region that works overtime is the area responsible for bringing negative *feelings* into consciousness. *These feelings can be completely fabricated: they do not need to have occurred in reality!*

- All of these different brain areas are connected by neural pathways – so when one is activated, the others are also stimulated. *What happens ultimately is that when a sad emotion is made conscious, old memories of sad events that match the feeling are whipped up too.*

- Because the brain is 'turned in on itself', the depressed person cannot concentrate on anything else and is locked into the gloominess. *This explains why depressed people seem to fixate abnormally on their intensely negative emotional state.*

One of the ways that antidepressant medications work is by 'switching on' neurotransmitters in the brain that are underactive.

Once the adrenaline has bounced against the hypothalamus to elicit its response, these little adrenaline 'balls' are broken down and eliminated because they are no longer needed. More adrenaline will only be produced if needed for another adrenalin surge.

Serotonin is another neurotransmitter, and has tempering qualities. Think of it as consisting of little capsules of 'calming potion' – not sedative, but calming.

DR DORA: Serotonin and stress

From a psychiatric point of view, the link between serotonin and 'stress' is indirect and complicated. Research has shown that low serotonin levels promote aggression, violent suicide and poor impulse control. For example, a man who suddenly decides to commit suicide (impulsively) by shooting himself (aggressive act) will probably have low brain serotonin levels.[18]

In addition, serotonin is actually indirectly implicated in anxiety. Rather than being a 'calming' neurotransmitter in these parts of the brain, it can even *promote* anxiety. Excessive serotonin in certain brain areas causes various anxiety disorders, particularly panic attacks.[19]

But for the moment, let us concentrate on the areas in which low serotonin levels can be associated with depression. When the little serotonin capsules are released from their serotonin nerve, they travel to the hypothalamus. As these capsules bounce against the hypothalamus, they deliver the 'tempering' potion to the hypothalamus, eliciting the response of emotional control, along with the adrenaline which is being 'felt' at the other end of the hypothalamus.

The serotonin nerve produces its little serotonin 'balls' in small amounts when there is a small amount of 'tempering' to do, for instance, to relax one before bedtime. It also produces a larger amount of serotonin balls when a huge amount of wellbeing takes place, for instance falling in love! It's one of the reasons why newlyweds behave like such soppy, rubbery fools all the time – believe me, I've been through it.

DR DORA: Serotonin in the human brain

Serotonin is a neurotransmitter that keeps popping up regardless of which psychiatric field is studied. It is implicated in:

- depression
- anxiety
- aggression
- sleep
- suicide
- sexuality
- being 'out of touch with reality' (psychosis).

Psychiatrists are not the only ones fascinated with this molecule: other medical specialists study its role in migraine, Alzheimer's, pain control, blood pressure and temperature, breathing and heart rate.

There are several problems with the serotonin hypothesis of depression:

- Serotonin does not act *alone* in any of the above conditions. It is far too simplistic to say that the model of serotonin underactivity or overactivity is responsible for depression. In fact, low serotonin levels are found in at least 10 other serious illnesses of the brain and nervous system.
- In addition, serotonin always affects other neurotransmitters. Every time serotonin levels increase or decrease, there is a cascade of other neurotransmitters that are similarly affected.
- It is very hard to measure how serotonin levels change during depression and its treatment. Scientists have only very indirect methods available to them. In other words, there is no 'blood test' for depression or any other psychiatric condition.

Despite its essential role in psychiatry, less than 1% of the body's serotonin is found in the brain! Most of it is in platelets (a type of blood cell) and the gut. To make matters even more complicated, there are over 20 types of 'locks' – called receptors – that the serotonin 'key' can fit into, each of which has a different function and effect on the brain. So, it is a very complex scenario within the brain, a lot more so than we are mentioning here, in order for you to understand a small amount about this incredible organ!

Adrenaline and serotonin are produced constantly in small amounts, as needed, and then sucked back into their reuptake sites for recycling. The thing is, they never actually work alone. When serotonin is released in small amounts, there is also a small amount of adrenaline being produced. This is not to prevent us from sleeping, for instance, but it does temper the serotonin enough so that we don't fall over with the first yawn.

In the same way, if a lot of adrenaline is produced, like when you are confronted by a dangerous criminal, for instance, your hypothalamus translates the signals into physical reactions of stress: sweating, panic, alertness, etc. But at the same time, serotonin is also released in fairly large quantities to 'temper' the adrenaline. This serotonin moderates the response to enable you to act appropriately. It does not 'relax' you into offering the assailant a cup of tea and a biscuit, but 'controls' or 'tempers' the adrenaline surge and transforms it into workable action in a way that helps you decide what action is best to take, e.g.: 'I won't scream uncontrollably. I'll do as I'm told but will try to move carefully towards the panic button to alert the security company, then try and negotiate with this man and see whether or not I can keep myself out of danger.'

Try and remember this example when your mind starts thinking of serotonin as an 'opponent' to adrenaline. It doesn't oppose it so much as direct and control it into acting more specifically and effectively. So, adrenaline and serotonin need each other to work correctly, and thus are released at the same time as each other.

So, once the serotonin capsules have been released, the empty capsules need to be recycled. The body is a very environmentally friendly creature, you see. So, these capsules get sucked back up into the serotonin nerve, by means of a reuptake site. Much like the 'out' and 'in' doors of a restaurant kitchen operate. Just like a waiter emerges from the kitchen with a plate of food, delivers it to you, and then goes back into the kitchen through another door to get the next load of food; so the serotonin capsules come out of the serotonin nerve to deliver the potion to the hypothalamus, and then return through another door, to get 'reloaded'.

A problem can arise, however, which tends to change things a bit. Sometimes, in some people, the reuptake site for the serotonin capsules is too efficient. In fact, it is trying so hard to recycle everything that it actually sucks the serotonin capsules back into the nerve before they have delivered their message! In other words, the serotonin nerve is producing plenty of serotonin, in lovely little capsules, which pop out of one end of the nerve, hoping to deliver their packages of control to the hypothalamus, but never get there! They are instead recycled all beautifully and efficiently, but without having actually delivered their message to hypothalamus! The result? A hypothalamus which is receiving normal messages from adrenaline, and waiting to hear the messages from serotonin, but never actually does.

Some people have a fairly strong adrenalin/serotonin imbalance, and have somehow learnt to cope with it very admirably. They feel permanently 'uptight' for little or no reason at all. They are alert and driven, and yet this drive is often not controlled; it results in them feeling desperately anxious about all problems, big and small, and they do not seem to be able to 'relax and put it into perspective', because their bodies keep experiencing the fight-or-flight response. The strange thing is that many of these people aren't even aware that the consequences of this imbalance are abnormal. They live with this ongoing struggle, in the genuine belief that everyone else feels the same, and that they simply 'aren't as good as everyone else' at coping.

DR DORA: The complexity of mood control

Control of mood is extremely complicated. We have already discussed several factors that play an essential role. Let us begin by ruling out environment, personality, genetics and electrical activity of the brain, as well as hormones. We will focus only on *neurotransmitter function* for the purpose of this discussion.

To explain the complexity of mood control, let us use the analogy of an orchestra playing a symphony. Imagine an orchestra of many different instruments. Each instrument is a different neurotransmitter. The music you hear is the dominant mood. Serotonin and adrenaline are just two of many 'instruments' (the violin and flute, say). They do have an effect on the symphony, or mood. But when you hear them play alone, they do not give the full tune. Only when all the instruments play together is the symphony heard.

Imagine that the conductor of the orchestra represents the emotional centre of the brain – the limbic system. Each instrument influences the conductor and s/he influences the playing of the instrument by waving a baton. But does the conductor directly cause the instrument's sound? Not at all: there are many other factors that come between the sound made and the conductor's baton. In the same way, in the human brain, there is no strict cause and effect. For example, serotonergic neurons do not connect directly with the hypothalamus to modulate emotional responses.

Similarly, individual neurotransmitters have some effect on the limbic system but they do not control emotion on their own. In different areas, they have different effects. Sometimes the same neurotransmitter will have *opposite* effects on mood, depending where it acts! In addition, serotonin and adrenaline interact with each other like two instruments. When one plays loudly, the other plays loudly. They also cause all the other 'instruments' around them to play differently. Bear this complexity in mind as we continue!

DR DORA: What is going on with serotonin and adrenaline?

From a very simplistic point of view, high adrenaline levels (in certain brain areas and under certain conditions) promote anxiety. But we throw a spanner in the works of simplified understanding, by noting that high levels of serotonin are also linked to anxiety symptoms! When the levels of these two neurotransmitters are low, depression predominates. This equation does not explain fully *why depression and anxiety so frequently co-exist*. You can see the danger here of simple explanations! They tend to lead us to oversimplified conclusions.

Traditionally, depression and anxiety were viewed as entirely different conditions requiring different treatment. There are some people who still hold this view, but it remains controversial.[20] Although the causes of the two disorders are *different*, treatment strategies that work for one frequently work for the other. In fact, it is hard to tease depression and anxiety apart.

- In predominantly anxious patients, depression occurs in at least 50% of cases.[21] There is such an overlap that some researchers regard depression as a *complication* of long-term anxiety.[22]
- Panic disorder is a very serious anxiety disorder that is disabling and terrifying. People suffering from panic are often depressed and are at a higher risk for suicide than people who are simply depressed or anxious.[23]
- When depressed patients have co-existing anxiety, they tend to be more severely ill, stay ill for longer and have a weaker response to antidepressant medication.[24]

I like to use the following analogy to describe what a clinical depressive may feel like. Consider the way you feel after a big fright, like a serious car accident, but one in which no-one was hurt. Perhaps the following emotions and experiences would be present, as they are in a clinical depressive, to a greater or lesser extent depending on the severity of the disorder:

- a feeling that 'it is all a bit too much to cope with'
- disorderly, 'swimming' thoughts; nothing cohesive or structured
- difficulty in bringing to mind small things such as your telephone number or street address
- irritability and defensiveness
- anger and short-temperedness
- intermittent heart palpitations
- a very twisted tummy, butterflies and extreme discomfort (like a spastic colon)
- tremors and shakiness
- rapid and short breathing, including hyperventilation

- light-headedness and slight nausea
- a sense of impending doom

...and then for quite some time afterwards:

- lowered defences to cope with what else may arise
- emotion and possibly tearfulness at the slightest provocation, even if unrelated
- ongoing guilt
- lowered self-esteem and feelings of worthlessness
- a need to 'curl up into a ball and hope that everything will go away'
- a low libido!

The initial symptoms immediately after the accident are all as a result of adrenaline overload. They are natural, and will pass. The problem arises when some or many of the above sensations are 'normal' parts of your day-to-day living, regardless of whether or not anything as extreme as an accident has occurred. This inappropriate response indicates not an adrenaline overload, but 'untempered' adrenaline. You may feel as though you have more adrenaline than other people do. You probably don't. It just feels like it because none of the adrenaline is being tempered or controlled properly. And this is called persistent anxiety.

The secondary symptoms to the 'car accident' scenario persist for much longer than perhaps would seem appropriate. When you try to reason with yourself, or when people tell you to get a grip on yourself, not only are you unable to do so, but this action in itself actually aggravates these symptoms, and tends to make you feel out of control. This may well be indicative of clinical depression.

The way I normally pick up that somebody may have anxiety and/or clinical depression is if they come to me for nutritional advice to find out why their energy levels are so low, and to find out if I can cure their lethargy. Now, I am not for one moment suggesting that lethargy always indicates a psychiatric disorder and that the patient must automatically be treated by a psychiatrist. Very often the problem is a result of incorrect eating habits, in which case an appropriate diet easily corrects the cause, and I never see the patient again (a success in our practice).

I am, however, referring to the fact that many patients have been living with the problem for so long that they have learnt to cope, and feel that 'this is just the way things are'. But frequently this perpetual lethargy is accompanied by some or all of the other symptoms of depression:

- an increased reliance on a diary, as short-term memory seems a bit poor
- irritability, and unexplained anger and tears
- extreme difficulty in getting up in the morning
- irrational nervousness about projects and goals
- poor self-esteem
- a feeling of not being able to cope; hopelessness
- ongoing feelings of anxiety and guilt
- decreased libido
- changes in sleep patterns; sleeping too much, or insomnia and night wakes
- changes in eating habits; appetite too high or too low
- changes in weight; sudden and unexplained losses or gains
- feelings of panic, inappropriate fear of impending doom.

These are feelings we probably all experience in our day-to-day lives, but with most people they go away as soon as the stressor causing them has been dealt with. One step further, and we may simply be going through a stressed time at work or at home, which may also pass and be forgotten, not yielding any further problems. One step further on from this, and we have an ongoing 'nagging' of all the above feelings, for no real reason.

This is medically termed dysthymia, and psychologists consider it to be serious enough to warrant therapy. This is because they know that if not dealt with properly, the problem can become more serious. They also recommend therapy at this point, because sometimes the stressor is something that won't go away.

DR DORA: Dysthymia

There are other forms of depressed mood identified by the American Psychiatric Association, such as *dysthymia*.[25] This is a form of chronic, low-grade depression that lasts for at least two years. In addition to the feeling of depression, there may be sleep disturbance (too little or too much sleep); poor appetite or overeating; low energy; low self esteem; poor concentration and feelings of hopelessness. Like major depression, dysthymia is more common in women than men. It seems to be on the spectrum of mood disorders and is less severe than major depression.

DR DORA: Adjusting to loss

Bereavement should not be confused with depression, although the normal reaction after the death of a loved one is very similar to depression. A grieving person experiences terrible sadness, frequently has insomnia, poor appetite and weight loss. These symptoms usually cease after two months. Certain symptoms are more characteristic of depression than of mourning and may point to a diagnosis of major depression. These include excessive guilt, persistent thoughts of death or suicide, feelings of worthlessness, markedly slowed movements and inability to function.

Sometimes, a very stressful event can cause behavioural changes that resemble depression. This is called an *'adjustment disorder'* in the DSM-IV.[26] Emotional and behavioural responses must occur within three months of the stress. Typically, there is weepiness and some of the physical features of major depression too.

If the stressor that is causing the problem has gone, and it has caused an impact greater than that which can be coped with alone, then this does not signify weakness. It is almost impossible for us to deal with some things alone.

For example, to deal with my practice, I wish to concentrate on being the best dietician I can. So I devote all of my time to doing research, seeing patients, reading the latest info from around the world, cooking up a storm with Kosher food, Halaal foods, fat-free Christmas dinners, and party food that a desperate mother had need of immediately for her diabetic child's birthday. It is for this reason that I have the professionals around to cope with things that I'm sure I could cope with, but choose to leave to the experts, who I know won't make a mistake. These are my accountant, my banker, my GP, my domestic worker, my electrician, my computer wizard, my receptionist, Patricia, who somehow acts like 15 people all at once, and so on. Even this book has been handed over to an editor who has put all my thoughts into sentences that are suitable for public consumption! All these people serve their purposes, and I find that the more professionals there are available to do what they are trained to do best, the quicker, smoother and more easily the intricacies of a practice are managed.

Yes, I probably could cope on my own, as I did when I was starting up the practice, but boy, was it an ongoing effort – constantly floundering around, buying self-help accounting books that I couldn't get through because my account was about to drop into overdraft if I didn't spend the time working to bring it up again. I could go on boring you with my mundane beginnings, but the point I am trying to make is that if there is something that needs to be sorted out, go to the expert, and get some trained advice on coping mechanisms. It may not be all quick and simple, but consider how long the problem would linger without a trained professional's help!

What's more, a professional will not keep you for another six months if s/he assesses that the problem does not need further treatment – they're all too overworked to do this. So, if you think there may be a need for a psychologist, then go! Only two things can happen: s/he tells you that you really do not need help – you are just worrying too much and everything will be fine if you stop watching horror movies; or you both find out that something can be done, and the therapist knows just how to do it. What bliss!

I'll bet you are wondering if I see a 'shrink' or not. Of course – upon the recommendation of a good friend, who saw me after a hard day with particularly worrying patients and told me that I need someone else who isn't inside this troubled and distressed mind of mine, to help me organise my concerns into a more organised and productive framework. Thank heavens! For what I thought were just temporary apprehensions about difficult patients were actually signs that I needed a break, and soon! Without her having told me that from an outsider's view, I would have continued on my merry way, and pent up all this anxiety to suddenly explode at some innocent bystander who took the last of the fat free cream cheeses at the supermarket.

DR DORA: Psychotherapy – who should go?

The 'talking cure' has been around in various forms for centuries. In the 19th century, there was an explosion of interest in the mind, its disorders and how to treat them. Two hundred years later, we have many schools of psychotherapy.

It is difficult to study how effective therapy is as a treatment tool, because so many therapies depend on things that are hard to quantify. The personality of the therapist is one such factor: it's essential but how is it measured? Ultimately, the relationship that develops between client and therapist is a strong predictor of whether the therapy will work, but it is almost impossible to measure! A good 'match', with chemistry and rapport, is more important than the specific school the therapist belong to. When it comes to treating most cases of anxiety and depression, a *combination* of psychotherapy and medication seems to work best.

Should people who are not clinically depressed see therapists? This depends on individual preference. It can be very useful to understand the factors underlying one's behaviour, especially when specific patterns keep recurring. Ideally, therapy provides some sort of insight into why we behave the way we do and gives us tools to act differently ... easier said than done!

This clinical depression can kill. Yes, it is a lethal disorder, which, left untreated, can lead to eventual organ dysfunction and death (a heart attack, for instance), or psychiatric-related death, such as nervous breakdown and suicide. Many people hear this and automatically shriek, saying, 'I'm not going to kill myself!', as if because they are not that sick yet, they don't have clinical depression at all. This is like saying, 'Because I do not need to go to hospital for pneumonia, I therefore do not have flu.' Depression may be there, in its early stages, and if left untreated can eventually reach a level of disastrous severity. This is why it is important for people to know exactly how dangerous a disease it is.

All the symptoms discussed already also relate to simple stress. However, persistent anxiety, as it is often called, is pathological, in that it can gradually destroy the body and its organs. Now, destruction is not just a bout of stress, is it? It occurs when a state of anxiety is prolonged without cessation. It is when the body enters the resistance phase of stress. This can be an unusually long period of life stressors, such as a traumatic family situation, or an unhealthy work environment. And because the resistance phase is long, the body passes through stages 1, 2 and 3, entering the conversion phase of stress, into distress and disease.

Some instances are stressful enough, and occur for a long enough period of time to create an organic (or physical) change in the activities of the brain chemicals. Again, the psychological effects of such situations need treatment, because there is only so much a human being can deal with alone, but that is the mind issue and a psychologist's help is needed.

The brain issue is what I am discussing, here. It is the physical alteration of brain chemicals that have caused other physical or organic changes to take place in the rest of the body. And because these symptoms or changes in the body are chronic (they persist over a long period of time, regardless of the environment), they become debilitating to the person inside that body. This is when the problem is a disorder or a disease: when it is no longer just unpleasant, but actually prevents you from living your life in a normal, healthy manner.

What is 'healthy', then? I know that 'healthy' can mean different things to different people, depending on their expectations of life. But I like the yardstick by which the great Freud himself measured it. He said that someone has true mental health if they are able to live, love and work. If any of these are suffering because of the symptoms mentioned above, then chances are you need an assessment for an underlying disease, such as depression.

Life is always going to be filled with misfortune, unhappiness, difficulty and extremely trying circumstances. Some people even believe that these horrible parts of life are sent to us for a reason. So do I. But no matter what you believe, 'shit happens', and you can't escape life's little knocks. What you can do, however, is battle through them with strength, courage and hope, and come out the other side stronger and more able to deal with them next time they arise. If you are one of the millions who feel the symptoms of stress, regardless of when the stressor is removed, and even after taking all necessary measures to get yourself 'back up' again, then the problem is probably organic, not psychological.

We were put here to do some good and to contribute to the greater scheme of things. If this seems like a daunting task, then assess why, for heavens' sake. Why do you feel as though you haven't enough to give? Is it because you believe what your negative mind is telling you over and over again, or is it because there are chemicals in there, whose balance isn't quite right?

Whatever the problem might be, solve it! You can't carry on taking and not giving anything back! You were put here for a purpose. Now find it, and carry it out!

Sometimes this really does make a depressive feel bad. S/he feels guilty for not knowing what it is s/he should do, as well as feeling guilty for not actually having the energy to carry it through successfully. If you really have tried, and tried again to do everything in your power to be happier, more energetic or more positive, and still you feel only transient improvements in your chutzpah, you ought to see a professional.

Again, I see the clinical depressives and those with persistent anxiety wince. I have hit a nerve. After all, isn't this the control freak who relies so heavily on adrenaline? Isn't this the person who has succeeded for so long, despite these well-hidden feelings of persistent anxiety? Isn't this the person who knows that everyone else seems to take things in their stride without showing any of the anxiety that is quietly crippling her? Aren't you the one who has spent your whole life carefully cultivating this high-powered 'in control' exterior, whose trembling and frightened child inside cannot possibly be seen?

I know what you may be thinking, then: 'Don't you dare try and expose my fear inside: I will defend my dignity with as much aggression as I need to. After all, no one else is so weak inside, are they?'

The truth? Of course everyone is! Everyone in this world has a frightened child inside of him or her. It is what makes the 'powerful' CEO sing too loudly in the car, with complete relief, after a good business deal. Or makes the marketing manager snap angrily when someone asks a question whose answer he does not know. We are all scared. In people whose serotonin works OK, the calming potion is released along with the burst of adrenaline, and it doesn't harm our brains or bodies. But in someone whose serotonin function is depressed, the adrenaline signal carries on a lot longer, with more intensity, and usually to the detriment of the depressive or those around him or her. This detrimental effect is what drives the nail deeper into the individual's guilt and chisels further into his or her dwindling self-esteem or sense of control.

So, you can see how debilitating this is, especially since the depressive often thinks that life is like this for everyone, but that everyone else has more strength and control. How demeaning can this be to one human being? Especially one whose serotonin can't even wash over and bring wellbeing (hard though it may be trying to).

And you know how hard you can be on yourself. Feelings of worthlessness only serve to spiral downwards, and you begin disbelieving all compliments (thinking that they are transparent lies to try and make you feel better), and internalising all well-meant criticism.

The criticism to which I am referring comes from everyone who is around you, who eventually exclaims: 'Just take a chill pill! Nothing is that bad,' or, 'Why can't you just snap out of it?' or, 'You're over-reacting and falling apart at the seams. Pull yourself together, now.' Just consider what this does to the soul. You may already be painfully aware that your coping skills are not as strong as they should be, but cannot understand why. Now you are getting a scolding which you believe is deserved, and so it is internalised. This obviously stimulates a fresh wave of adrenaline production ... need I say more?

Years of this, and you will be an exhausted wreck of nerves. And it's ongoing. It doesn't stop when you are 'relaxed'. You have no chemical means by which to relax! People with many psychiatric disorders live like this 24 hours a day, and somehow manage to carry on without many of us thinking more about them than that they are just 'nervy' people. Talk about swimming upstream!

Other problems of the clinically depressed

Are these people OK? I think it depends on what you call OK. They may function adequately, but their poor self-esteem is crippling and inescapable, inside. They truly believe that they are a waste of space. And their defensiveness and hopelessness take more energy out of them each minute than a day of white water rafting takes out of Joe Bloggs. Now tell me if they are OK. No wonder they have a host of other problems that constantly niggle at their already broken sense of wellbeing:

- water retention
- stubborn weight changes
- spastic colon
- hormonal changes, causing increased body odour, acne, unusual hair growth, changes in menstrual cycle, and many others
- repeated sore throats, thrush, ear infections, coughs, colds and flu at the drop of a hat, and unknown viruses
- allergies to random factors; post-nasal drip, eczema, asthma, psoriasis, etc.

Are they OK? I think not. And just think of the money they have to cough up at every visit to the various practitioners who are so specialised that they don't often think to look at the bigger picture.

Sometimes, however, practitioners do prescribe the correct treatment for this diagnosis, only to be automatically stonewalled as the patient's already turbulent mind conjures up horror stories of sedation, straightjackets and men in white coats. They harbour feelings of betrayal towards their trusted practitioner, as if the doctor is trying to prove to them that they are too weak to cope alone. And a perfectly appropriate diagnosis and treatment fly out of the window, whilst paranoia seeps through the adrenaline-swamped grey matter.

And all because of a stigma attached by ignorant know-it-alls.

After the above little scenario the clinical depressive will, in a split second, deduce that the GP s/he has trusted for 35 years has had enough of the ongoing problems and is now out to make money out of the family. The decision to prescribe an anti-depressant has turned the kind, caring and trusted practitioner into a drug-wielding fiend who will, from this moment forth, laugh at every weakness and try to administer every pill possible to keep the 'hypochondriac' quiet.

But – have you ever thought that perhaps the anti-antidepressant women's magazines might be wrong, and the GP might actually be right?

Never! is triumphantly sounded, and off to the naturopath, homeopath, or dietician you traipse. The pendulum has swung from pure faith in medicine to a hatred of anything textbook or mainstream. The individual lands at my clinic, demanding healing for the lethargy with anything it takes, but not drugs.

I am left helpless! Contrary to popular opinion, a dietician's job is by no means naturopathic or 'alternative'. We are medical school-trained professionals, whose job is to assess nutritional diseases and treat them or to adjust nutritional prescriptions according to the disease at hand. We are not people who try and cure disease using 'natural' foodstuffs or vitamins without drug intervention! So, I am left with an unhappy patient, who thinks that now the world is trying to sedate him/her into oblivion, when all that is wanted is a little more energy!

But psychiatric disorders are diseases of the brain, which is only an organ, just like your leg, or skin! They are debilitating. By debilitating, I mean they prevent you from being you, and push you into a spiralling cycle of events; feeling less and less able to cope, which makes you push yourself harder, which serves to highlight your decreased productivity, which worsens your feelings of guilt, which lowers your self-esteem, which makes you more irritable and despondent, which further serves to convince you that there really isn't much to live for after all.

Stop! You are unwell! You need treatment, and fast!

I have seen this spiralling of events in patients who are convinced that there is nothing wrong with them at all and deny their disorder, seeking the help of all sorts of alternative healers and trying to take endless quantities of vitamin tonics for energy. Though many of these alternative therapies serve to improve the symptoms, they are not dealing with the disease: a simple chemical imbalance.

OK, you must be thinking, how can we tell the difference between a psychological problem and a chemical one? How do you know whether or not the problem is for a psychologist or a psychiatrist? More often than not, it is a problem for both. But let's get to differentiating a little, here.

Most people think that psychologists are for people who are flaky and wear funny clothes. People also think that psychiatrists are for loonies, and that the treatment they offer consists exclusively of popping their victims into a straightjacket for life and frying their brain with endless electro-shock therapies. Wrong! Of course, these practices are used when other methods do not work for people with really severe psychiatric disorders that are life-threatening and untreatable. The rest of the time treatment is highly specialised, dealing with common problems that 'normal' people have, for which a psychologist is inappropriate or insufficient.

Let's get back to the differences here and use an inextricably South African analogy. If you were part of an armed hold-up in a bank, and the shock thereafter caused your personality and actions to change, then you may have post-traumatic stress disorder (PTSD). This ongoing fear of guns, being attacked, and constant bad and violent dreams would definitely warrant the help of a psychologist. He/she would talk you through the mental anguish you have experienced, and work to formulate skills to overcome your phobias. Without that therapist you probably would be scarred for life, and never quite be the same again. But voilà! Help worked!

If you were in this situation, however, and following this, you noticed the above symptoms of clinical depression starting to be continuous, then chances are it's not necessarily your mind's thoughts that have been affected, but the chemicals inside your brain. In the same way as somebody who has lost their oestrogen as a result of a total hysterectomy, you have an imbalance of hormones, which will bring about certain changes in your body and brain. The only way to restore the original function will be to replace the missing hormone with hormone replacement therapy.

The same applies to the chemicals or neurotransmitters in the brain. If there is a physical imbalance of the brain chemicals' activities, then no matter how skilled the psychologist is, no matter how much therapy you get, those chemicals probably won't change. So, it is not a mental thing, it is a chemical thing. And the only person equipped to deal with this chemical imbalance is one who has studied only this for 12 years or more at medical school – a psychiatrist!

DR DORA: What is the difference between a psychologist and psychiatrist?

Many people get confused between the two disciplines of psychology and psychiatry. *Psychiatrists* are medical doctors who specialise in mental illness. This is much in the same way that surgeons specialise in performing operations. Psychiatrists are therefore trained to pick up neurological or medical problems. In addition, they can prescribe medication. Many psychiatrists also treat patients with psychotherapy.

Psychologists do not undergo medical training. Rather, they are specialists in performing psychotherapy (for individuals, groups or couples). They are also able to administer 'psychometric tests'. These tests allow them to describe a person's psychological profile.

So, getting back to who should treat the condition, the psychiatrist will have all the skills and knowledge to be able to assess the problem specifically, will be able to ascertain exactly what treatment to give you, and then will probably suggest appropriate medication which best deals with the problem and the person who is experiencing it – you. Unfortunately, like any diet, there is no easy one-formula-fits-all for treating clinical depression, and that is why you will want a trained expert to be as specific as possible, for the most effective outcome. The thing is, however, that the psychiatrist will usually recommend psychotherapy as well, to help you cope with the mental anguish the depression has led you to experience, and to help pick up the pieces and get you back to being your well, productive and happy self again.

The golden rule to remember, though, is that these professionals are not mind-readers. They need you to tell them exactly what is going on, and you must want them to treat you. They will not treat you if you are not willing. And this is why I am writing this book, to take away the 'stigma' that appears to be attached to mental ill-health. If there is a problem, acknowledge it, and use the people that are there, and who know all about it. You'll never look back.

Again, several years ago there was an attitude towards people with diabetes. It was taboo to even think of that poor person injecting himself three times a day! That was when people were ignorant about the disease. No longer is he 'that man who is dependent on drugs'. People have been educated to understand that he is not strange or dependent on drugs. He is simply replacing what his body cannot produce!

The same applies to clinical depression. The patient probably has more than enough serotonin, but it just functions very irregularly. So, the way to fix it is to know what is happening in that magnificent and hidden brain of ours. We simply help the brain function the way it was born to. One of the most recent discoveries was that of the selective serotonin reuptake inhibitors (SSRIs). These simply sit in the reuptake (or recycling) site of the serotonin nerve, and prevent the serotonin that is released from being 'sucked back' up again. All they do, in fact, is allow the serotonin that your body is wanting to release (the amount depends on how you, as an individual, reacts to things) to do its job.

That is, it returns you to the person that your genes wanted you to be: whether that be nutty, emotional, reactive or just plain boring. But this time, you will be reacting to each circumstance in your own individual way, in a way that you feel is controllable, doesn't seem too much to cope with and is not inappropriate. You will also be much nicer to your kids, your husband, even your pets. And to yourself. And if there are psychological matters to be dealt with, you will now be in a clear and perky position to work through them, and succeed with greater ease.

DR DORA: Medications used in treating depression

People have used natural remedies for depression throughout history; but only in the last 150 years have new treatments been synthesised and studied. In 1955, some patients were being treated for tuberculosis with a drug called isoniazid. The TB didn't get much better, but the patients became euphoric! So, the first 'happiness' drug had been discovered. Three years later, the tricyclic antidepressants, a new class, were identified. Since then, there has been a mushrooming of interest and activity in developing better, safer, 'cleaner' antidepressants with fewer side effects. Drugs are no longer stumbled across through serendipity; rather they are designed to target specific areas of the nerves. They play a refined role in the neurotransmitter pathways. The selective serotonin reuptake inhibitors (SSRIs) prevent serotonin being pumped back into the neuron for recycling; so the amount of serotonin available is increased. Newer drugs inhibit the reuptake of both serotonin and adrenaline, which sounds as though it may defeat the object, but actually serves to control the balance of production. Others have effects on specific receptors, so they act indirectly on neurotransmission. Despite all the marketing, no single antidepressant has been shown to be more effective than the old tricyclics. These drugs, unfortunately, have many side-effects so they are used less and less, but they remain the gold standard of treatment.

SSRIs and other anti-depressants don't take away your problems, and they don't make you happy. In fact, people who are being successfully treated for depression actually say they now feel everything much, much more acutely, and are more able to cope with life in the way they know they should. They say that clinical depression made them 'numb' to all feelings except despondency, and now they are able to cry harder, laugh harder, and sit quieter than they ever thought possible. It makes the problems that are dealt with much more real, but they are now in the same frame of mind as with Joe Bloggs next door, who is able to become anxious about a problem, deal with it to the best of his ability, and then forget about it once it is done.

It sounds obvious, but it is incredible how the press has given anti-depressants such a bad name, through ignorance, that the clinical depression sufferer refuses to acknowledge that s/he may suffer, for blind fear of such ridicule! It is only through ignorance that this is even said, and hopefully awareness will increase so that the little pill taken every morning will be as accepted as the injection taken by insulin-dependent diabetics.

I truly do not think that it is at all fair for some journalists and features editors to spout forth with words holier than thou about how depression need not be treated with drugs. I mean, firstly, who are they to be so knowledgeable about clinical depression? The very fact they make such flippant comments probably means that they have never met anyone with clinical depression, or think that they have gone through a 'nasty time' themselves, and have come out of it using a course in découpage. What they are getting confused about is the word 'depression'.

Yes, we all feel depressed at times. Often, in fact, if we live in the city! But this is by no means anything like clinical depression. No ma'am. It is not classified as a psychiatric disorder for fun, and people do not spend millions each year on a miraculous 'happy' pill which will somehow take away their problems. This must be one of the most dangerous misconceptions ever, and prevents people from taking anti-depressants, in favour of some perceived martyrdom. Martyrdom is for things we, as humans, have the power to stand up to. Anti-depressants are for diseases which are organic in nature, and which we know usually get worse without them. Just like a paraplegic cannot just 'get up and sort herself out', neither can a clinical depressive 'just snap out of it, and see the wood for the trees'. Because that's one of the jobs of serotonin, and believe me, no one wants that balance more than a clinical depressive.

DR DORA: What can an antidepressant do for you?

Many people I see in my practice are frightened of using antidepressants. They have heard stories about 'addiction', 'personality change' and 'emotional numbing'. There are many myths around about antidepressants, so let's use this opportunity to address each one.

- **Antidepressants are addictive.** There is no scientific evidence that antidepressants are addictive. The same dose can be used in a patient, for decades, without the body becoming used to it. There is no 'withdrawal reaction' or craving when an antidepressant is stopped. However, many doctors recommend that the patient should be slowly withdrawn from an antidepressant to prevent relapse of depression. Very occasionally, antidepressants with a short 'half life' are used. This term means that the particular drug does not last long in the body. When it is suddenly stopped, the patient may experience mild withdrawal-like symptoms.

- **Antidepressants change your personality.** Again, there is no evidence of this. No drugs have been developed that 'change personality'! All antidepressants do is make your mood happier and calmer. On average, a person taking antidepressants should feel content – *not* euphoric.

- **Antidepressants make you emotionally numb.** Not at all. A depression can make you indifferent to the world and your future; not the treatment! When a person is on antidepressants, there is an improvement in baseline mood, as mentioned above. In addition, if something tragic happens, of course, the person responds with grief. If an amazing event occurs, the person will feel happy.

- **So, where do these myths come from?** It is true that antidepressants are widely prescribed. If they are prescribed wisely for the correct indication, they work well. It is when they are used for the wrong reasons that they cause problems or do not work. The 'horror stories' one reads in sensational newspapers and magazines have never been proven in the scientific literature. But they cause a lot of damage and turn people against safe, effective medication that can save lives!

Many people are curious to know why clinical depression is so prevalent now.

1. Is it a new fad that people are using as a crutch for not being able to pull themselves together?
2. Is it that a new wave of ethno-bongo hippies are trying to make everyone have the same personalities, and not allow people to be themselves, even if some people are a bit unpleasant to be with, or seem a bit aggressive?
3. Isn't it just that I'm going through a rough patch, and that a good holiday will sort me out?
4. Surely I don't have a chemical imbalance! I'm just an uptight sort of person!
5. My adrenaline is what got me where I am today! You can't take it away!
6. I was in the Second World War, and I don't need drugs or therapy! Why now does this new generation seem to pop pills for everything that goes wrong?
7. There's a pill for every ill. Why don't people just accept that they aren't the 'copers' in life, and carry on with a brave face?
8. Why is it that so many people suffer from this depression thing, but when I was growing up, it wasn't something that was even heard of!

I would like to give a response to each and every one of these comments, and by doing so, will further highlight exactly why each statement is made out of ignorance and is not true.

But first I will retell a story to dispel such ignorant banter. A 24-year-old man was improving on a daily basis, on anti-depressants, and his family was thrilled to know that this life-long problem had been identified, and he was returning back to his old self after 10 or so years of anguish. All until a friend noticed that he was on antidepressants, and told him that he was mad to be on those things. Didn't he know that they are very addictive? Didn't he know that he must just get a new job and kick out that girlfriend, and everything will fall into place? You don't need those things, man, you're not mad! So he came off them out of complete despair. Eight weeks later he shot himself in the head.

If that young chap hadn't tried to play psychiatrist, and if social stigmas weren't so crooked, he would still be with us.

1. If clinical depressives could pull themselves together, they would! They, of all people, are the most strong-willed people you know! If they weren't they wouldn't have lasted for so long! People who have recovered from clinical depression often succeed well beyond their wildest dreams. This is because they had learnt to keep up with the rest of us, whilst suffering through all that anxiety. They say it was almost like swimming upstream. Now their depression is controlled, they actually have a head start with respect to stamina! Never tell someone to pull themselves together, unless it is just a silly spell!

2. A clinical depressive's personality is not showing up! Their problem is! It is like saying that someone who is under anaesthetic must have a very low IQ. Rubbish! Their altered state has changed them! It is chemicals we are talking about, here, not personalities. Besides, once clinical depression has been controlled, the person's personality won't change! He will simply be more himself! If that personality is naturally grumpy and aggressive, so be it. But whilst he is under the control of haywire adrenaline, by no means is he himself!

3. Clinical depression is basically chemical. Going away on holiday may relieve some of the symptoms, simply because the body isn't producing as much adrenaline. But return to the day-to-day hurdles that are a natural part of life, and the problems arise. You cannot keep hoping that the problem will go away once this is over, or once that has been sorted out. There will always be problems, and if your responses to them are inappropriate, deal with it!

4. If you are a naturally uptight person, then genetics are to be accepted and loved as they are. But if there appear to be problems that are making it difficult for you to function as you know you should, then that 'uptightness' needs to be sorted out.

5. Clinical depression is often hereditary. If one or more of your parents had it, then there is about a 15% chance that you have it, too. If you were born with it, then you may have lived your life with a nagging suspicion that you can't cope with things as well as your peers. By this, I don't mean you couldn't keep up! You simply noticed that you always did the things that they did, but it was always with an extra dose of anxiety and intensity. Because of this, you may have made it a subconscious goal to always do just a little bit better than anyone else, to retain your pride and hide your feelings of inadequacy, even though nobody even knew about them! Although the adrenaline always made you a little more anxious than everyone else seemed to be, the good thing is that it kept you awake late into the night when that project needed to be better than everyone else's. That adrenaline gave you the drive to keep going, to be a perfectionist, to be an all-or-nothing person that got you where you are today. But no one said anything about taking away your adrenaline! Medication will simply temper it to a usable, productive source, one that will no longer be complicated with feelings of hyperanxiety, worthlessness and exhaustion, but rather with the serotonin directing it towards whatever goals you have chosen! SSRIs do not work on the adrenaline, remember? They only help serotonin work to direct it effectively!

6. Listen up, old chap! We respect you because you risked your life for us all. But you can't simply turn a stiff upper lip to what has happened in your body's chemical make up! If trauma like that hasn't affected you at all, then you really are very lucky. But for the many, many people who suffer from post-traumatic stress disorder, turning a stiff upper lip to the problem may wreak havoc. The poor victim may suffer both mentally and physically from psychological damage as well as chemical imbalance. This stiff upper lip attitude may lead to a silent and unspoken acceptance of a life of nightmares, stomach disorders, alcohol abuse, withdrawal from society, severe emotional outbursts, diminished sexual performance and general disquiet within himself. He may have retained his dignity with the chaps at the club, but the personal life he has to keep so secret has silently decayed into one that is fairly lonely and unhappy.

7. O.K., we can all just accept our shortcomings, and take on less. But isn't that like telling a diabetic that he should just accept that he has a disorder, not rely on drugs, and take the rough with the smooth, even if that means losing his sight and limbs? Possibly even his life? But diabetes is a life-threatening disease, you exclaim! So is depression. Why else would a person take his or her life? Because there is no other way out of such despair. Don't underestimate depression. If untreated, depression kills. But if treated correctly, there is no worry at all. A GP I work closely with says that depression is one of the most fascinating diseases she knows, and the most rewarding. This, she says, is because it can kill. But on the other hand, the treatment of the disease results in such dramatic improvements in a matter of weeks, that the patient's relief at returning to 'themselves' again is all the high a GP needs!

8. The truth is, some people have always suffered from, or carried the potential for clinical depression throughout the ages. But they were the ones people dropped their eyes for when discussing them, because they either drank themselves into a coma, committed suicide, or were thrown into a loony bin and sedated when they became too much to handle. Thank God we understand it now! That is why it appears that so many people are suddenly afflicted with this 'new' disease. We can now diagnose them successfully, and treat them so that they can continue running the company we work for, and continue to provide us with their individual skills and talents!

Clinical depression can also be described as something which may be carried, latently. For instance, we now know that cancer has a genetic basis. So, if someone carrying a cancer gene were to live 1000 years ago, with nothing more to worry about than whether or not the sun would rise, and he lived on fresh veggies, didn't drink vodka or sit in a tense, airconditioned office, but in the depths of the Fertile Crescent, and smoking was something that fires did, then chances are that cancer would remain latent, and never make him sick. If, however, that same person with the same genes was put in Johannesburg right now, the anxiety, the pollution, the alcohol excesses, the smoking and the perpetual threat for one's life would definitely lead to that gene rearing its ugly head, and causing cancer of some sort.

Likewise, in our ancestors, whose adrenaline level's biggest surge was in response to the fact that the bread didn't rise adequately, the genes for depression may not have been forced into activation. But

I need not go into what we all experience in our day-to-day modern lives for you to appreciate that the ongoing stressors we are subjected to mean that those people carrying a genetic predisposition to clinical depression will stand a very good chance of becoming actively ill.

These days, there are more particular stressors that can also bring on an increased occurrence of the disorder. Those like an unrealistic goal for body weight, for instance. Not only is this enough of a stressor to bring on depression, if given enough importance in a genetically predisposed person's mind. The other, additional danger is that the actual calorie restricting to get there induces its own chemical imbalances, leading to clinical depression.

If, somehow, the stigma of psychiatric illness could be removed completely, many of us practitioners would be able to do our jobs so much more quickly and efficiently and there would be fewer tired people in the world. You see, many, many people are still living in the shuttered 17th century when it comes to psychiatry. Mention the practitioner's profession, and you conjure up long halls of disturbed people wandering around in their own world. Yes, there are people in the world who are that sick, and most of them are not frightening at all. Just very sick.

But for the rest of the world, many of whom are unknowingly suffering from clinical depression and persistent anxiety, psychiatry is precisely what is needed to sort the chemical imbalance out, once and for all, and the long halls and white coats don't even come into it. Left undiagnosed or untreated, this problem can manifest itself in many parts of our lives, systematically ruining all that we hold dear, like a healthy and slim body ...

4 THE HPA AXIS

In the previous chapter we saw how an imbalance in brain chemicals causes persistent anxiety. This chapter will examine the way clinical depression affects other parts of the body.

The human brain is quite magnificent. It turns sensory perceptions such as sight, touch (pain, heat), smell and hearing into conscious experiences, then, through the hypothalamus, translates this conscious thought into an emotional and physical response by means of a hormonal reaction throughout the body. This chapter will examine this process – which includes, but also goes far beyond, the function of adrenaline and serotonin already discussed. Once you understand this process, the far-reaching physical implications of clinical depression will be evident, as well as how little depression actually has to do with feeling sad, and how physical the symptoms – many of which you may well recognise – are.

The hypothalamus translates thought into an emotional response, in addition to three other functions:

- It produces hormones (ADH and oxytocin) to regulate blood pressure and activate sexual function, respectively. In clinical depression and persistent anxiety, disturbances in the production of this anti-diuretic hormone (ADH), lead to significant water retention, which is often treated singularly with diuretics. Unfortunately, this forces the body to change a symptom rather than treating the underlying depression or anxiety. As a result of a forced feedback mechanism from the drug, the patient is now rendered dependent on such diuretics, and the problem is only worsened.

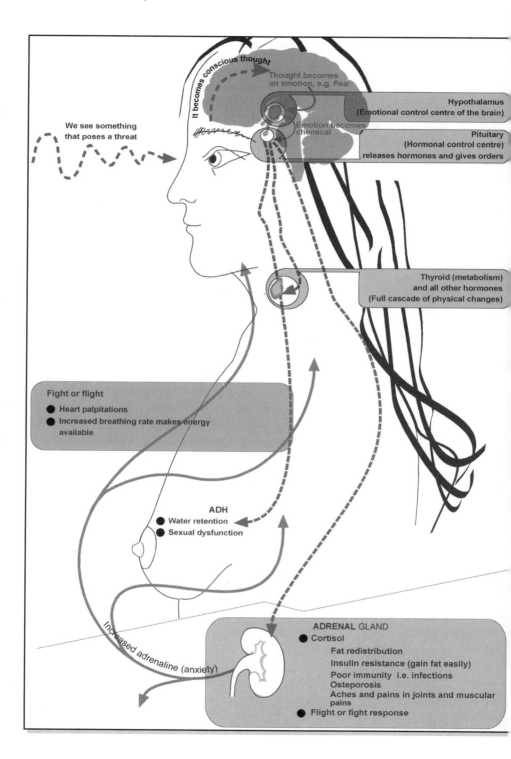

- It signals to the pituitary, the 'control room' for most other hormones in the body, which is situated just below the hypothalamus. In this way, conscious thought becomes emotions, which become physical actions or symptoms, many of which are accentuated in anxiety disorders.
- It signals to the adrenal glands, which sit on top of the kidneys, to produce adrenaline, to actually activate the complete physical fight-or-flight response. (At the same time, it receives input from serotonin.)

And you thought clinical depression was only psychological? Read on. The following details about hormones and their functions will help you understand the mechanisms involved and how extensive the symptoms of clinical depression are. So, follow me into the labyrinth of hormonal function in the human body, and just watch in amazement while we uncover some of the mysteries underlying this misunderstood condition. Please don't expect to remember it all afterwards – I am not giving you a crash course in physiology! If you merely understand it, then I have done my job. Once you realise how someone with depression is suffering from overwhelming physical as well as mental discomfort, then you can start appreciating how 'irritating character traits' may in fact be symptoms of physical disease.

The HPA axis sounds like some enemy coalition out to fight the allied forces. But it is nothing of the sort! It is a medical term for the hormonal integration system, which controls a surprisingly large portion of our beings. It stands for the glands which secrete the hormones responsible for most of the activities in our bodies, namely the hypothalamus, the pituitary and the adrenal glands. It is named as such because it is an interlinked axis of control mechanisms. These mechanisms are disturbed in clinical depression, which explains how an imbalance in the adrenaline-serotonin function can cause all the other seemingly unrelated problems – the general malaise by which we are confounded.

We have briefly discussed the hypothalamus being the 'processor of thought into emotions and hormones, so now let's move on.

The pituitary gland

Situated below the hypothalamus is the pituitary gland. They say that dynamite comes in small packages, and biology proves this point.

This small gland is about the size of a marble, and yet it controls all of the following processes (in fact, while you read, you may recognise many symptoms you had no idea were related to anxiety and stress, so heed well, so that you can start understanding your body's cries of exhaustion):

- thyroid-stimulating hormone (TSH) – controlling the thyroid and metabolism
- adrenocorticotropic hormone (ACTH) – directly controlling the 'fight-or-flight' response from the adrenal glands
- follicle-stimulating hormone (FSH) – controlling the sex hormones and fertility
- luteinising hormone (LH) – ovulation in women and testosterone production in males
- prolactin (PRL) – controlling activities in the breast tissue of women
- growth hormone (GH) – controlling growth and fat and protein metabolism
- melanocyte-stimulating hormone (MSH) – controlling the pigment in the skin
- anti-diuretic hormone (ADH) – controlling blood pressure and bodily fluid regulation
- oxytocin (OT) – controlling milk production in women and sperm regulation in men.

As you can see, it really does regulate nearly all of the body's functioning! Let's talk about those functions which are directly relevant to this book:

Growth hormone production

Growth hormone is responsible for breaking down fats and muscle in the body (auto-cannibalising) for the liver to use as sugar for energy in the blood. In clinical depression, this production is often altered. Since clinical depression is an ongoing and inappropriate stress, growth hormone is continually active in an attempt to fill the blood with sugar for use by the muscles to either fight or flee. Though there is no reason to run from today's stress, because there is no physical danger, the brain feels the fight-or-flight response with its unopposed adrenaline and noradrenaline, and interprets this as danger.

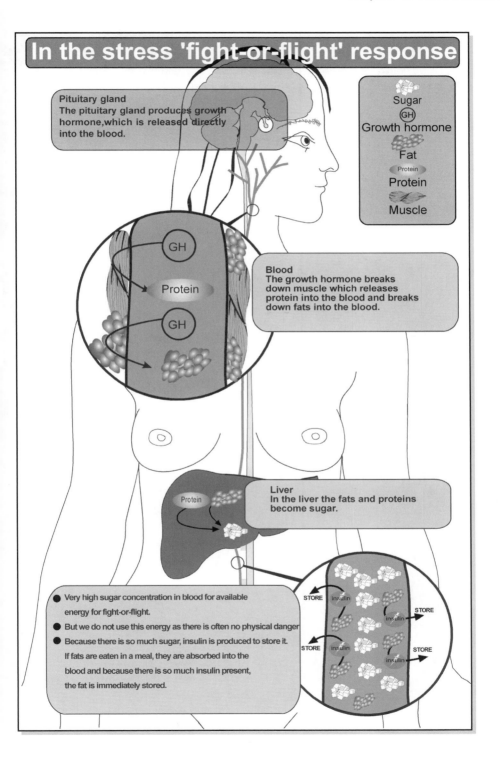

In the stress 'fight-or-flight' response

Pituitary gland
The pituitary gland produces growth hormone, which is released directly into the blood.

Sugar
Growth hormone
Fat
Protein
Muscle

Blood
The growth hormone breaks down muscle which releases protein into the blood and breaks down fats into the blood.

Liver
In the liver the fats and proteins become sugar.

● Very high sugar concentration in blood for available energy for fight-or-flight.

● But we do not use this energy as there is often no physical danger

● Because there is so much sugar, insulin is produced to store it. If fats are eaten in a meal, they are absorbed into the blood and because there is so much insulin present, the fat is immediately stored.

Although the blood is continuously flooded with sugar, hardly any of it is used for the intended purpose: fight or flight. Consequently, there are large amounts of sugar in the blood and an increased insulin production to try and store that sugar. This process mimics diabetes. This 'diabetic' effect automatically induces storage mode, which causes rapid fat gain and consequent difficult fat loss. The body fat-muscle proportions will also change: the process of auto-cannibalisation reduces muscle mass and thus metabolism, and consequently the fat percentage increases. This change induces a state of even further insulin resistance, and is a major cause of Syndrome X and its symptoms – obesity, diabetes, hypertension, high cholesterol, etc. (see *The X Diet).*

DR DORA: Growth hormone in depression

Growth hormone does exactly that: it helps the body grow. Normally, it is secreted in little spurts at night. It makes sense that young children and adolescents secrete more growth hormone than the elderly. In *depressed* people, secretion of this hormone is increased but it occurs during the day, rather than at night.[1] In fact, too little growth hormone is produced at night.[2] It has been suggested that *disturbed sleep architecture* is what causes the diminished growth hormone release.

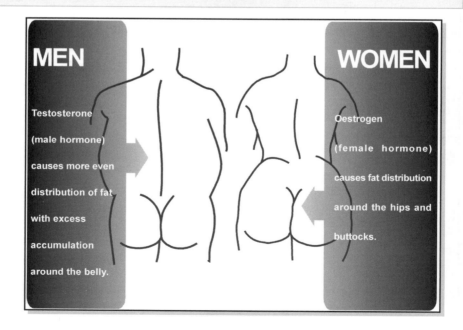

MEN

Testosterone

(male hormone)

causes more even

distribution of fat

with excess

accumulation

around the belly.

WOMEN

Oestrogen

(female hormone)

causes fat distribution

around the hips and

buttocks.

Not only do clinical depressives experience difficulty in maintaining control of the psyche, they find it equally difficult to maintain control of a previously well-preserved physique. The contrary can also happen, though. Some individuals will lose weight during clinical depression. This very much depends on which phase of the generalised adaptation state (GAS) they are in: the alarm phase, in which case they will lose weight quickly, or the resistance and exhaustion phases, during which their body is much more in the mode of 'storage' for preservation, and they will gain weight.

Prolactin release

Prolactin is released from the pituitary gland. When a woman gives birth, this hormone stimulates lactation, or breastfeeding. (It is also present in men, but the function is largely unknown, apart from being partially involved in the production of the male hormones, androgens.)

When a new mother suffers from post-natal depression, the production of prolactin may decrease from the levels needed in lactation, preventing her from breast-feeding. The necessity for an anti-depressant during post-natal depression is rarely disputed, because the symptoms are so pronounced, sudden and obvious. The reason for this will be explored later on in the book, when we discuss female hormones.

However, in non-pregnant depressive states, the production of prolactin may in fact be significantly elevated. This is very common indeed, and causes swelling in the breast areas of both men and women, as well as altered sex hormone production. This hyperprolactinaemia (hyper – too much, prolactin – the hormone; aemia – in the blood) leads to changes in body composition, impotence in males, infertility in women, and a host of other HPA axis problems. It can be very easily diagnosed and treated, but can, itself, also bring on symptoms of a more prolific problem, such as depression. Hyperprolactinaemia can also lead to rapid and unexplained weight gain.

Activation of sex hormones

The sex hormones are activated by the pituitary gland. These hormones induce the desire to make love and are responsible for the reproductive cycle and fertility. In clinical depression, the first notable symptom is often poor libido and inability to have an orgasm in women, and impotence in men, as a result of these altered hormones.

There is an increase in cortisol production (see below) in anxiety and depressive states, and this decreases the production of the sex hormones. Not only can this interfere with sexual function, but it also worsens the pre-existing loss of libido that is so common in depressed people.

Unfortunately, sexual dysfunction is still a largely taboo topic and is not often raised in the practitioner's office. Decrease in libido is often attributed to age, a failing marriage (although this in itself can be a result of the sexual dysfunction) or other emotional reasons, when actually it can improve significantly if the underlying component is addressed, namely the depression or stress disorder.

Furthermore, many secondary problems may arise from other hormonal dysfunctions, such as polycystic ovarian syndrome. This can be exacerbated as a result of the insulin resistance caused by the growth hormone's 'diabetic' effect. (See below for more about this.) Endometriosis has also been closely linked with clinical depression, due to the altered female and male hormone production. In both cases, infertility may result, causing further anxiety to the clinical depressive. Finally, if the female sufferer is approaching the exhaustion phase of the generalised adaptation state, then she will stop having periods altogether. This is not only a result of anorexia nervosa, but also of the stress response in clinical depression.

Polycystic ovarian syndrome

by Drs Jacobson, Kuchenbecker and Gobetz (info@vitalab.com)

Polycystic ovarian syndrome (PCOS) is a common condition occurring in one out of every nine women of the reproductive age group. It is characterised by an abnormal hormone function that leads to excessive androgen production by the ovaries. This results in abnormal ovarian function and various effects on other body systems. PCOS is a heterogeneous condition with some women presenting with severe symptoms and others only having minimal complaints. This disease cannot be cured but timely management can limit its implications. Many women with mild to moderate disease are not diagnosed and thus denied the opportunity to limit the short and long-term implications of PCOS. It is therefore important for all women to be aware of this condition and to seek medical advice.

A basic understanding of the mechanism and control of ovulation is essential in order to understand the nature of PCOS. The pituitary gland produces hormones called follicle stimulating hormone

(FSH) and luteinising hormone (LH) which control the ovulatory cycle. As the menstrual period begins, FSH stimulates the growth and development of a follicle. A midcycle rise in the LH matures the egg and leads to ovulation 24-36 hours later. This normally occurs 14 days before the onset of the next menstrual period in those women with normal menstrual cycles. The developing egg secretes oestrogen which stimulates the lining of the womb (endometrium) to grow. The cells surrounding the follicle produce androgens in response to LH. These minimal amounts of androgens are essential for normal egg development and ovulation. After ovulation, the remains of the follicle secrete progesterone, a hormone that finally prepares the womb for a possible pregnancy. If fertilisation does not occur, secretion of oestrogen and progesterone by the follicle ceases with a decline of hormonal support of the endometrium. This is followed by the onset of the menstrual period. A delicate interaction between the ovary and the pituitary gland controls the ovulatory and menstrual cycle.

Although not yet well understood, research indicates that an abnormal function of the enzymes that control the ovarian hormone production leads to PCOS. A genetic link explains the clustering of PCOS in certain families. This enzyme abnormality results in a high concentration of androgens being produced in the ovary with resulting poor egg development and absence of ovulation. This disruption of the ovarian function leads to the formation of multiple small follicles in the ovary that fail to mature and ovulate. The androgens also enter the blood circulation with the following effects on the rest of the body.

- An abnormal feedback mechanism between the ovary and the pituitary gland leads to the excessive production of LH which in turn stimulates more androgen production in the ovaries, initiating a vicious cycle of events.
- The androgens react with receptors in the skin resulting in male pattern hair growth, acne and in severe cases even male pattern baldness.
- Androgens are also converted to estrogens in fatty tissue resulting in high blood level of oestrogens.

Resistance of various body tissues to the effect of insulin is another important factor associated with PCOS. This resistance leads to high blood levels of insulin, which, together with other related substances, stimulate the production of androgens in the ovaries. The resistance to insulin is enhanced and aggravated by obesity, which thus increases the signs and symptoms of PCOS.

Some patients complain of minimal symptoms while others present with a severe disease. The following symptoms may be indicative of PCOS:

- Menstrual irregularities are the most common symptom of PCOS. These can vary from mild irregularity of the periods to excessive menses, to total absence of menstruation for prolonged periods of time.
- PCOS is inevitably associated with infertility because of the inefficiency and/or absence of the ovulatory process. A previous pregnancy does not exclude underlying PCOS because the expression of PCOS may have been initiated by an increase in body weight after the pregnancy.
- Male pattern hair growth, acne and in severe cases male pattern baldness may be an expression of the high blood levels of androgens in patients with PCOS. These symptoms vary according to the individual sensitivity of the skin tissue to androgens. Genetic predisposition and the ethnic origin of the patient may influence this sensitivity to androgens. Women of Mediterranean origin tend to have a high skin sensitivity to androgens, while Asian and Scandinavian women might not have any symptoms in spite of high circulating androgen levels.
- Spontaneous miscarriage occurs more commonly in patients with PCOS, most probably due to high blood levels of LH and inadequate production of progesterone to support an early pregnancy.
- Obesity is a factor commonly associated with PCOS and it may aggravate the condition. It is however not a prerequisite for the diagnosis. These patients often experience difficulty in losing weight in spite of dietary efforts.

The abnormal blood lipid profile associated with PCOS as well as obesity and insulin resistance increases the risk for high blood pressure, heart vessel disease and diabetes. High circulating oestrogen over a prolonged period of time initiates excessive stimulation and growth of the endometrium. This growth is not opposed and balanced by progesterone on a regular basis because of the absence of ovulation and thus leads to proliferative growth on the endometrium and an increased risk of endometrial cancer.

Women with the above symptoms should undergo a thorough assessment by a gynaecologist. Women whose mothers had PCOS should carefully watch for these symptoms and seek help if they develop any of the signs or symptoms. PCOS patients with female children should inform their children that they are at risk and watch for symptoms. Menstrual irregularity after puberty could be an early indication of PCOS and intervention at this stage could prevent excessive male pattern hair growth and thus avoid long-term cosmetic effects.

A thorough medical history and physical examination by a gynaecologist will indicate the extent of the disease and this baseline assessment is essential to monitor the response of treatment. Blood tests should be performed not only to diagnose PCOS, but also to exclude other hormonal problems that may mimic the symptoms of PCOS, like abnormal prolactin production or a dysfunction of the adrenal gland. An increased LH/FSH hormone ratio as well as a raised free androgen level in the blood is suggestive and most often diagnostic of PCOS. In the setting of the symptoms of PCOS, the diagnosis can best be confirmed by the typical appearance of the ovaries on ultrasound.

The high incidence of insulin resistance and risk of developing frank diabetes necessitates testing of the fasting insulin and glucose level. After the menopause these women are still at increased risk of developing diabetes and heart vessel disease. Regular assessment of the blood pressure, fasting glucose and cholesterol will allow the early detection of disease and enable management that will contain progression of these problems. Sampling of the endometrium is indicated in patients with very few or absence of menstruation in order to exclude early premalignant change.

Cortisol production

The pituitary gland controls the production of cortisol from the adrenal glands. Cortisol is a stress hormone which is released in the fight-or-flight response. It enables the body to mobilise energy for use during the stress phase. Unfortunately, however, this is where things start to go 'wrong', as regards the physical effects of long-term stress and depression. This is one of the major reasons why we gain fat so rapidly during phases of increased stress and distress.

When the stress response begins, the pituitary signals to the adrenal glands to produce cortisol. For instance, if a tiger is chasing you, the pituitary signals for the release of cortisol to mobilise energy for running away from it or fighting it. The bloodstream fills with cortisol, and the brain registers that the blood now has sufficient levels for the action. It can tell this because there are little sensors in the pituitary which monitor the blood for how much cortisol has actually been released, and whether or not it is sufficient. When these sensors receive the signals from the cortisol in the blood, they signal the adrenal glands to stop producing any more. If running from the tiger is not successful, then the pituitary again signals to the adrenals to produce more cortisol, as the response must be continued. Again, it signals this production until it senses that enough has been released into the bloodstream, and then it stops signalling. Usually this is enough for you to be able to remove yourself from the stress. In this case, cortisol has done its job and stops being produced.

Unfortunately (or fortunately!), there are no tigers in the workplace, and so the stress is often not something we can run from and alleviate in a matter of minutes. So the stress response continues, and the bloodstream is continually filled with cortisol, which is never 'used'. The sensors in the pituitary keep sensing the high levels, and yet the pituitary has to keep producing more, because the stress response never lets up. As a result, the pituitary sensors start ignoring the continual notification of a high blood cortisol level, and stop indicating to the brain that there is a lot of cortisol floating around.

So, after ongoing stressful situations, the pituitary has got 'used to' a high cortisol level in the blood, and stops noticing it. The result is that the pituitary loses its ability to actively stop the cortisol production when the stressor is removed (you go on holiday or finish a project, but you cannot relax). This high level of cortisol in the blood, even after the stressor has gone, indicates a disturbance in the HPA axis, and depression or persistent anxiety. It is a good example of the 'conversion reaction' we discussed in chapter 2. Something that has been stressful for too long has actually forced you to become adapted to this state, and you have developed a chronic disease as a result.

Cortisol not only contributes to this mental stress response, but also to the physical symptoms of weight gain, water retention, insulin resistance and susceptibility to infections and disease. It also initiates the 'diabetic' effect, auto-cannibalising the fat and muscle tissue to enable the liver to produce new sugar for the blood. It causes insulin resistance, causing the clinical depressive to gain fat very quickly and lose it with great difficulty.

To understand how cortisol functions in depression (because it is overproduced), compare what happens to a person who receives cortisone treatment for eczema, transplants or severe allergies. (Cortisone is the same stuff as cortisol, it is just what is medicated, rather than being produced by our own bodies.) Such a person will tend to gain fat very quickly and find it difficult to lose, regardless of effort. Weight control becomes almost impossible. Moreover, the individual will retain a lot of water, and the fat stores tend to move away from the hips and thighs to settle around the midriff as well as the face and neck. This change in body fat distribution is also concurrent with insulin resistance and Syndrome X, and thus carries the additional potential for heart disease and diabetes.

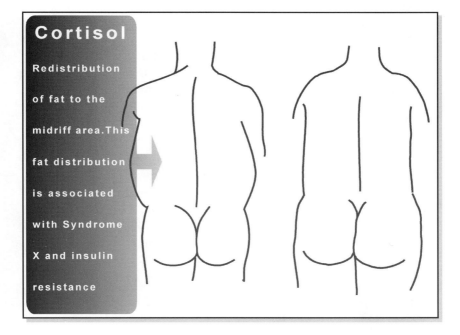

Cortisol

Redistribution of fat to the midriff area. This fat distribution is associated with Syndrome X and insulin resistance

When clinical depression causes elevated cortisol levels, the body's inflammatory responses are blunted. This serves a purpose in trauma or real short-term stress situations, when the body needs energy for running and fighting, not inflammation.

Another downside of elevated cortisol levels is poor immunity, causing heightened susceptibility to many infections and diseases that the body would under normal circumstances easily fight. The most common ailments clinical depressives suffer from are upper respiratory tract infections (URTIs). What's more, the individual may have persistent underlying infections – never quite bad enough to warrant a trip to the doctor, however. Although these underlying infections do not make you feel obviously ill, in some ways they are worse than a full-blown infection, because they destroy the body's immunity.

These minor infections remove the iron in the blood that carries oxygen to the cells for normal metabolism and energy production. Most infections 'feed off' iron to survive, and to prevent the infection from proliferating, the body removes iron from the blood and stores it in the liver, in an effort to 'starve' the infection. It is often very effective in doing just this, and helping to eliminate the infection, but the result is a mildly anaemic clinical depressive – just to add insult to injury.

The physical lethargy brought about by iron depletion often warrants a visit to the doctor. However, very often iron supplementation is recommended, without examining any underlying reasons for this anaemia. This directly worsens the problem, because increasing the iron intake (by either food or supplementation) simply feeds the infection what it needs, and encourages the infection to prevail!

It is important to treat the infection with antibiotics, because often in a stressful situation, the body's defence mechanism is so compromised that antibiotics are the only way to get rid of it. It is, however, vital to establish why the infection occurred in the first place. Because the human body is so incredibly well equipped to deal with most disease, especially minor infections, when such an infection occurs, it usually indicates that something else is wrong. Furthermore, the body responds to getting sick by depressing serotonin production, exacerbating the clinical depression and compromising the body's ability to heal.

DR DORA: The HPA axis: stress and depression

Whenever we are faced with a real or a perceived danger, the body primes itself to respond. A cascade of events occurs which culminates in the secretion of the stress hormones. These stress hormones get the body's sugars and fats broken down for quick access to energy. Other hormones in the stress response stop the body doing 'non-essential' things like growing and reproducing, in order to conserve energy. The brain instructs the adrenal glands to pump out adrenaline to prepare the heart and muscles for action.

- Information about the dangerous situation reaches the hypothalamus, which is under the control of various neurotransmitters such as serotonin and adrenaline, among others.

- The hypothalamus secretes hormones that stimulate the next part of the chain, the pituitary. The most important of these is called *corticotropin releasing factor* (CRF). Remember CRF, because we will be examining how it contributes to depression, further on.

- The pituitary then sends a hormone messenger to the adrenal glands, causing them to secrete cortisol.

- In depression, the adrenal glands are on emergency standby to secrete floods of cortisol. They are hyperactive and supersensitive, even if the signal to secrete is a small one.

- When depression is successfully treated, these hormonal abnormalities disappear.[3]

- For the sake of accuracy, please note that the pituitary's releasing hormone is not the only stimulus for cortisol production. It is more complicated than this, but we will keep it simple for clarity.

- Also, high cortisol levels occur in many other conditions besides depression (anorexia, alcoholism, malnutrition, dementia).

For the last 40 years, evidence has accumulated that depressed people have a malfunction of their HPA axis. In depression, too much of the stress hormone, cortisol, is produced.[4-7] The more severe the depression, the higher the cortisol level.[8] Severely depressed people may ultimately take their lives. In suicide victims, cortisol levels are also increased on post mortem.[9]

One explanatory theory is that depressed people are suffering from *stress*. In a person who is genetically predisposed to developing depression, a stressful experience might precipitate a depressive episode. While there is some evidence that depressives are often exposed to high stress levels, this is *not always* true.

In depression, people often lose their appetite, in which case weight loss could account for the higher cortisol levels. Age also plays a role. The older the depressive, the more likely the increased cortisol level.[10]

In depressed people who are not on medication, CRF levels are high. After treatment, the levels drop. Certain experiments have given normal volunteers CRF directly into the central nervous system. The symptoms that follow are almost identical to depression: poor libido and appetite; sleep problems and sluggish movement. Responses similar to an acute stress reaction have also been described.[11] So, CRF may be producing many of the problems seen in depression and anxiety.

New treatments for depression are being studied all the time. One of these is a drug that opposes CRF in the body and counteracts its 'depression-producing' effects, although side-effects have been noted in many of these cases.

DR DORA: Stress and early experience of trauma — a fascinating field

Ever since the early theorists postulated that childhood trauma might reappear in adulthood as psychiatric illness, researchers have struggled to find proof. Now this is changing. There are exciting new developments in the field of hormone research which prove what many people have suspected all along. Early life stress and trauma may produce depression in later life. The main culprit seems to be CRF, the hypothalamic hormone that activates the stress response. Stress early in life makes the hypothalamic stress response *overactive*. Research has shown that this increased activity tends to persist into adulthood. The brain remains more sensitive to new stressful situations, frequently resulting in depression. Animal studies have proven this conclusively. In primates raised in a very stressful and unpredictable situation, there were elevated CRF levels in their central nervous systems, way down the line, in adulthood.[12] Similar results have been found in human studies. In sexually abused children, CRF levels were higher than in depressed children who were never abused.[13]

We know that childhood sexual abuse and neglect lead to increased rates of depression and anxiety later on in life.[14] This is particularly a problem for women, because girls experience sexual abuse more often than boys. The incidence varies from 6% to 62% of girls.[15] In South Africa, the incidence of child sexual abuse is high. In addition, other severe early traumas may increase the risk of psychiatric illness. As a child, if you lose a parent, have alcoholic, mentally ill or neglectful parents, or experience family violence, you may well be at risk for depression later on in adulthood.

Women are more vulnerable to depression than men. One reason may be that their HPA axes are more sensitive to stress, which results in depression later in life. Early experience of stress produces HPA hyperactivity. This is mediated by changes in the ways genes are read and expressed.[16] So, life experiences have an effect on the way our *genes* express themselves. The link here between stress, genetics and mood is the HPA axis.

Increased cortisol production contributes to many immunity problems, resulting in infections. However, some of the symptoms associated with simple infections are grossly misdiagnosed. A typical case of this is the 'fashionable' controversy surrounding candidiasis.

Misdiagnosing candidiasis

Clinical depression can also open the sufferer to long-term problems, such as ongoing vaginal thrush, or in extremely severe immune compromise, thrush on the tongue and fingernails.

Candidiasis is an infection of the external areas of the body, such as the vagina, by **Candida albicans** (a type of yeast). It occurs frequently in women whose homeostasis has been disturbed by certain drugs, the contraceptive pill, ongoing stress or other infections. Deep systemic candidiasis, however, is a very different condition, being manifested deep within the body's internal organs, and causing severe problems indeed, such as severe bloating, lethargy, irritability, allergies and so on. While you are reading these symptoms, you may well recognise them, and 'slot yourself' into the candidiasis category by virtue of the symptoms. But these are symptoms of exhaustion, stress, colds and flu, etc! They are not only those of deep candidiasis. Unfortunately, however, many patients are still incorrectly diagnosed with deep systemic candida, with their depressive symptoms being attributed to the infection. Real systemic candida, however, is very rare, and is usually only present after serious operative procedures, such as open heart surgery or transplants in infectious or unclean environments, or in severe immunocompromise, such as AIDS or cancer.

The minor vaginal candida invasion usually subsides rapidly after anti-depressive and standard nutritional treatment is commenced. By this, I mean following a low GI carbohydrate diet, which is low in fats, high in essential fatty acids, and rich in fruits, vegetables, salads and dairy products. The abovementioned misdiagnosis of candida is often treated with a standard 'candida diet'. This entails cutting out all wheat, yeast, mushrooms, acidic foods, sugar, preservatives, and dairy products. I must emphasise that this is not only unnecessary, but also dangerous, in light of how much of the healthy, prudent diet you are cutting out. You are relegated to leathery wheat-free bread, all foods devoid of wheat (including spices, many herbs, and so on ... the list is almost endless), and you are left with what? An anti-social and bland diet which is very difficult to fit into the prudent, low-fat high carbohydrate guidelines. And for what? The candida still recurs each and every time you have these foods in meals cooked by friends, and you start feeling as though you have an incurable disease which has left you incapable of enjoying life as you used to.

This candida diet was devised using many unscientific criteria. Firstly, if you had deep systemic candida, you would know that something was extremely wrong! You would find the infection in very obvious places; the nails, the tongue, the ears and the vagina. You would not need a diagnosis of something you cannot see; you would be in a very serious condition indeed. Candida infection of this kind literally starts damaging the internal organs, such as the liver, the bowels and the kidneys. This would lead to concurrent symptoms much more severe than the abovementioned few symptoms matching those of severe stress. If you have many complicated symptoms, such as white growths all over the tongue and nails, problems with urination, bladder infections, vaginal thrush, or if you have cancer, Aids, or have recently had open heart surgery in an unsterile environment, then you may need to see a GP about deep systemic candida.

Secondly, the diet prescribed is based on the following misconceptions: the fact that candida is a yeast does not mean that you must now avoid all types of yeast. This is like saying that since baboons are wild animals, then humans must be, too, because they are of the same zoological class! ***Candida albicans*** is in the same 'family' as brewer's yeast (used to make bread) – but it is not the same thing. Avoiding eating and drinking all yeasts is also futile: if candida has been able to infect the inside of the body it is because its spores floated there while the body cavity was open. Yeasts that are eaten cannot miraculously filter into the internal organs without being digested first! Suggesting that one should not inject yeasts directly into the bloodstream would be a more reasonable suggestion! Even then, this would bring about another set of problems, unrelated to the systemic infection, by virtue of the fact that it is a different organism entirely! The same misunderstanding leads to the suggestion of cutting out mushrooms! If mushrooms were the same as candida, then very bad vaginal thrush would be fairly visually frightening, need I say more ...?

Because the body's homeostasis can be altered by taking the contraceptive pill – which makes the vaginal secretions more acidic and therefore more easily infected by candida – the conclusion appears to have been made that all acidic foods should now be avoided. The blood's pH is so tightly controlled by the buffers in the blood, that food cannot have an effect on the internal environment, such as is suggested. Any change in pH within the body enough to cause an alteration in the blood's composition, would result in major problems, not just vaginal thrush. These would include cardiac arrest, dementia, radical hyperventilation and muscle tremors. The vaginal secretions become more acidic because the pill alters the composition of these fluids, not the blood! Eating acidic foods cannot have this effect, because the pH of the gastrointestinal fluids is more extreme than any foods we as humans could possibly manage. The pH of a lemon, for instance, is approximately 5.5. The pH of our stomach juices is approximately 3-4! Thus, at this stage of the GI tract, a lemon is seen as alkaline, not acidic! Our bodies are much cleverer than that!

Cutting out sugar is based on the half-understood concept that vaginal thrush grows well in a sugar-rich environment. If there is plenty of food, warmth, moisture and protection available (as in the vagina), then growth is optimised. Now we know that all carbohydrates are made up of sugar which dissolves into our bloodstream to carry energy to our cells. This blood will inevitably carry that sugar past the vessels in the vagina, thereby feeding the candida. So, it would seem logical to cut out all carbohydrates, right? Wrong!

Firstly, we must understand how each carbohydrate type dissolves into sugar at a different rate. This is called the Glycaemic Index. Those carbohydrates that dissolve into sugar quickly should be avoided, because they fill up the blood with sugar, thereby feeding the candida. However, suggesting that all carbohydrates be cut out not only defeats the object, but also starves the rest of your body, rendering it more helpless to fight against infection. This is why we use low GI carbohydrates to treat candida infections in the vagina. These fill the blood with sugar so marginally and slowly that the candida really does not have an optimum environment to live in – and if the rest of your body is well and fighting this infection, it will die off quite quickly.

So, this sounds as if it supports the very argument against eating refined sugar, right? Wrong again! Cane sugar is not a high GI carbohydrate! In fact, sugar has now been proven to have a medium GI, comparable to corn on the cob, rice and boiled potatoes. Again, people must be very careful about hanging onto simple words which are taken out of context by people who don't fully understand the concept themselves. 'Sugar' is a word describing the smallest component of a carbohydrate. We have in the past used it inappropriately to describe only one type of these sugars, namely sucrose, which still needs to be broken down into its component sugars, in order to filter into our blood. This process in sucrose is not immediate at all, as it is in glucose: it happens more slowly and reacts differently. The faulty conclusion, obviously, was drawn from that enemy of medical research: simple deduction. So, cutting out sugar is not only futile, but also allows us to ignore the 'real' high GI culprits: baked potatoes, rice crispies, maize meal, rice cakes, crispbreads and bread of all types.

This leads me to the last misconception. Bread has been blamed as an enemy of candida sufferers for several reasons. Firstly, because of the yeast content (as explained above); secondly because it is refined (another reason that is not a major factor in determining the GI of a carbohydrate), and finally, because it is wheat. The classic comment is, 'But when I cut out bread, my stomach stopped bloating!' If you had poor eyesight, which caused headaches, your symptoms would be worsened by a screaming baby, right? But the screaming baby isn't giving you that headache, it is only making it worse! Get glasses, and the screaming won't nearly be as bad.

This is just a silly example of how one can blame the wrong thing for a problem. The same holds for bread. Just because you may bloat after eating bread, it doesn't necessarily follow that you have candida or an allergy/intolerance to wheat! It is usually because of something much more underlying but more easily dealt with: a stress-induced spastic colon (irritable bowel syndrome). What's more, bread itself isn't even the problem: the type of fibre present is. You see, in irritable bowel syndrome (IBS), the stress response makes the colon too sensitive to what we call 'insoluble fibre'. This is the 'brown bits' you see in brown or wholewheat bread (which is always recommended as healthy). Now, although it is very healthy, people who suffer from stress and IBS will experience pain, bloating and irregular bowel movements when they have eaten this type of fibre. But it is not the wheat! It is the wholewheat! Eating other insoluble fibres, such as apples, guavas with their pips and beans will do the same to the stomach. This is by no means an allergy: it is a symptom that the stomach is being too sensitive to the stress response (whether it be stress, or an inappropriate anxiety condition).

With respect to food additives, the effect that these have on candida is negligible. If it is stress-related symptoms that are the problem, then dealing with the stress disorder will eliminate all symptoms within six weeks. If it is deep systemic candida, then hospitalised therapy needs to be initiated without hesitation, and a diet that is not only balanced but also highly nutritious. This is one of the most important aspects of the treatment of any immunity-related condition; cutting out preservatives is an unnecessary waste of time and energy.

An interesting fact discovered in recent years is that additives have an effect only on those people who are overtly allergic to such substances: asthmatics should avoid sodium benzoate and sulphur dioxide (SO_2), post-menopausal women with high blood pressure should avoid MSG, and the rest of us can relax, enjoy, and eat normal foods which our friends and family give us. In fact, tartrazine, once regarded as 'dangerous', has not only been conclusively proven to have no effect on hyperactivity, cancer or any other disease, but it has been suggested from the studies that it may even play a role in preventing cancer!

What I hope to have elucidated with all of this, is how easily complicated and unpleasant diets can be administered by unprofessional 'experts' who understand only some of the facts about nutrition.

And now back to cortisol ...

As we have seen, cortisol has an overt impact on our immunity, leading to minor infections such as candida, URTIs and mouth ulcers, all of which are easily overcome – for good – with the correct therapy.

One of the more unfortunate effects of depression-stimulated cortisol production is leaching of the bones. The elevated cortisol levels cause the bone to increase its turnover of minerals, mainly calcium, and thus more calcium is lost through the urine. Osteoporosis is very common in patients who have been treated with cortisone, and this may be a reason for poor bone density in depression.

Apart from the abovementioned compromised immunity symptoms, cortisol also has a role to play in insulin resistance. After prolonged stress, the body stops noticing the level of cortisol in the blood, and so the high cortisol levels become the 'norm'.

Cortisol stimulates the liver to produce and release glucose into the blood. It also inhibits the body's ability to obey insulin (thus 'insulin resistance'). Remember that insulin is released when our blood fills with sugar, so that it can store it into the muscles where it is needed for energy. Thus, as the body tries in vain to store sugar after a meal, it continues to produce ever more insulin, flooding the bloodstream. As if that were not enough, remember that insulin's role is to store! Anything! So, if your blood supply has an enormous amount of insulin in it, any fat that may be eaten in a meal (whether it be hidden or not) will be commanded very loudly, to get stored!

This is why people who are stressed, anxious and/or depressed can gain fat very easily. Moreover – eating less does not make it better, but worse! In fact, cortisol isn't the only thing that makes us insulin resistant: a high level of fats in the blood also makes us insulin resistant. So, if we eat a diet high in fat, we will become insulin resistant. When we reduce calories, however, the body empties fats into the bloodstream. This would seem a good thing, when we want to lose the stuff, but unfortunately, while losing some of it, the result is a bloodstream high in fat for some time, and ...insulin resistance!

Cortisol also decreases the amount of glucose used by the skin, as well as decreasing its oxygenation. This is why after prolonged stress, or in clinical depression, one's skin condition decreases dramatically.

Thyroid hormone production

The pituitary also regulates the production of thyroid hormones. The thyroid has gained all sorts of attention with the world-wide increase in obesity. In truth, the numbers of true hypothyroid sufferers who need medication are actually relatively small. The thyroid does control the metabolic output of energy in the body to a certain extent, but if the thyroid were the factor responsible for the onset of obesity, many other symptoms would present long before the onset of obesity. These are poor tolerance to cold, extreme lethargy, aching in the muscles and joints, dry skin, hair loss, slowed reflexes and puffiness under the skin. Having said this, these symptoms may well present alone, as hypothyroidism, where the thyroid gland is malfunctional. But the patient may simply have the condition as a result of the depression cascade effect on all other hormonal function.

The thyroid takes its signals from the pituitary gland, so if there is something wrong up there, then the thyroid may appear faulty. If thyroid hormones are then administered to correct this 'fault', then thyrotoxicosis may develop when the thyroid resumes normal activity every so often, giving the patient a 'double-whammy' of thyroid hormones! Often, the patient will have irregular thyroid measurements with different tests. This can be indicative of a secondary condition in addition to the clinical depression. Often hypothyroidism is diagnosed and treated without a comprehensive examination of underlying causes. Unfortunately, administering thyroid drugs will often exacerbate the anxiety, because thyroid hormones make the body even more sensitive to adrenaline.

DR DORA: Thyroid hormone and mood

When the thyroid gland produces too little thyroid hormone, the result looks very similar to depression. People suffering from an underactive thyroid gland complain of feeling weepy and exhausted. They have memory lapses and poor libido. Sound familiar? This has led to the hypothesis that in depression, there is abnormal control of thyroid gland by the hypothalamus.

Aldosterone production

The pituitary controls the production of aldosterone, which controls blood electrolytes. In clinical depression, however, this hormone may be inappropriately elevated at times. As a result, the patient's blood pressure starts rising. To make matters worse, the kidneys stop secreting salt to retain levels in the blood. To top it all, the taste buds for salt on the tongue become more active, thus increasing the need for and consumption of salty foods!

This hormone, aldosterone, can also be deficient in clinical depression. Again, this response depends on how the body reacts to the depression. If there is insufficient aldosterone production, the patient will feel light-headed and dizzy upon standing, and electrolytes will be lost extensively through the urine. The result is that the depressive also has poor nerve activity and can develop aches and pains in the muscles. Arthritis also develops through the kidney's inappropriate expulsion of metabolites.

Let's recap, to make sure you understand the process of clinical depression:

- The brain receives super-alert stress signals, because adrenaline is being produced (sadly, this happens often in this day and age). Serotonin is also being produced, but can't get its signal there.
- As a result, there is almost continuous 'super-anxiety'.
- Small tasks become daunting prospects, and the person will often procrastinate as an avoidance mechanism.
- Sleep is disturbed, and night wakes often occur at about 3 a.m. when the body's natural spurt of adrenaline and growth hormone takes place to rebuild the body. Normally, serotonin would be delivered as well to keep the sleeping process uninterrupted, but in this case, the person wakes up and cannot fall asleep again.
- Because the sleep is not serotonin-drenched, the person does not rest completely. Consequently, the person feels complete exhaustion and a sense of overwhelming impending doom during the day. (Remember that serotonin would allow just enough adrenaline to wake a person, not to cause a feeling of panic regarding the day.)
- The person will experience lethargy, moodiness, irritability, sometimes tearfulness, and defensiveness throughout the day.
- Productivity is decreased, and each task becomes a nerve-racking experience.
- Because of a change in appetite, the individual is drawn to snacking on junk food (sweets, chocolate, as well as coffee and cola to keep awake and replace the missing energy).
- Thoughts become jumbled, and short-term memory is compromised. As a result, the individual starts relying on a diary, because

all the information seems jumbled, rather than neatly catego-
rised in the brain.

- A pervasive sense of guilt is experienced, and the individual feels
worthless, with a sense of not being able to cope.
- Anxiety changes the bowel movement pattern, and alternating
constipation or mild diarrhoea can persist.
- Light-headedness and dizziness can occur, and blood pressure
may increase or decrease.
- Allergies such as nasal and sinus problems present themselves,
and skin changes can occur.
- Headaches are common, and migraine reactions occur more regularly.
- Minor infections, such as colds, sore throats, flu and bronchitis
begin.
- Weight starts to fluctuate, and although the need for exercise is
obvious, the individual is mostly too tired and would rather sleep
during any free time.
- There is a lack of interest in previously pleasurable activities, and
libido is compromised.
- In women the menstrual cycle is altered, along with fertility, and
in men problems with poor libido and impotence are rife. Water
retention and 'puffiness' is experienced, and the individual simply looks poorly.

This is clinical depression.

DR DORA: Is this chain of events what causes depression?

This model *explains* what happens in depression. In reality, the chain of events occur
simultaneously rather than sequentially. Remember that it is much more complicated: low
adrenalin levels are even associated with depression in certain brain areas! It is not clear
whether the high levels of stress hormones are the cause or effect of depression.

Of course most people will feel emotionally depressed with this level
of physical disruption! The irony is that this problem also often
manifests itself in people with 'Type A' personalities – those who are
instinctually driven to overachieve, succeed, control, be perfectionists, and to do things in an all-or-nothing manner. They are usually

the most angry when it appears that their bodies are 'failing' them, despite all their efforts to the contrary.

Many Type-A personalities have the desire to relax, but seem unable to do so. As a result, when these people suffer from depression, many turn to alcohol to 'switch off' adrenaline enough for them to feel 'normal' again, or drugs like Ecstasy and cocaine, to 'switch on' more serotonin. It is common for the depressive to have two or three drinks before being able to feel a little relaxed. To increase the feeling requires more alcohol, however. This soon leads to an unwitting increase in regular alcohol consumption, usually in greater quantities than normal, always in search of complete relaxation seemingly only achieved by drinking alcohol. Unfortunately, all of these substances only serve to increase the clinical depression once their immediate effect has worn off. As a result some depressives fall prey to drug and alcohol abuse simply to 'relax'.

The brain is a tangible, organic mass of nerves and connective tissue that both receives and sends chemicals and signals. The mind is the product of these chemical messages, producing intangible, abstract processes. In clinical depression this process goes awry. In order to understand these differences clearly, imagine losing someone close to you. Your mind goes through turmoil trying to understand, accept, and come to terms with the trauma. This is the psychological side of your brain in action. Your thoughts cause the turmoil or disturbances. In time, these disturbances should improve, especially if you go for psychotherapy.

The grief that is felt is overwhelming, but unfortunately it is very necessary to move through all its stages. This is when you should allow yourself to feel the pain, and allow full grieving, without taking any of it away. This is an appropriate response to psychological grief, painful though it may be. If, however, the psychological response to this loss does not improve over an extended period of time, then that person may need intensive psychological therapy, to help them move forward and regain their normal functioning in society. The help of a psychologist is called for, because the mind is not getting any better.

If this psychological pathology is severe enough, it can actually cause a disturbance within the chemicals of the brain. By this, I mean that thoughts have been so pathological (recurrent, intensive and ongoing), that the nerves within the brain have actually altered in their function. The problem is now psychiatric in nature. It has become physical, and affects organic parts of the body, not only the abstract, intangible thought processes of the mind. Since the problem is no longer only psychological, the therapy will be very difficult and frustrating indeed.

In the first instance a psychiatrist's intervention is required, to assess the physical problem of the brain chemicals; secondly a psychologist's intervention is required, to assess the patient's mental status. (Problems in this area may have been exacerbated by the psychological difficulties imposed by the psychiatric disorders.) This type of depression is caused by a psychological stimulus, which has become physical (psychiatric).

Hereditary clinical depression

There are many cases of clinical depression being idiopathic in nature (that is, of no known origin). This is most commonly hereditary clinical depression, meaning that the individual was born with a genetic predisposition to clinical depression.

A person suffering from hereditary clinical depression has a 15% chance of passing the disorder on to his/her offspring. This increases in cases where both parents carry the disorder. In the case of hereditary clinical depression, the individual may not experience the full extent of the disease until he or she is older, or unless a life-stress causes the onset.

Consider a genetic predisposition to breast cancer. If you are aware that you are carrying this gene, you have a choice, don't you? You could live carefully, take regular exercise, not smoke, drink alcohol in moderation, and follow a high-fibre, low fat diet. If you are lucky, the gene will remain inactive. However, should you choose an ill-advised lifestyle for one predisposed to cancer (no exercise, heavy smoking, eating fatty food, etc.) you stand a chance of activating the gene, and developing breast cancer.

The same exactly goes for the depressive predisposition. If that person's serotonin function is 'shaky' to begin with, then any situation that causes a dramatic increase in adrenaline production may suddenly bring to light the depression of serotonin function, where it had not really been an issue before. This is named the organ inferiority hypothesis, and describes how excessive stress will be reflected in damage to the weakest part of one's body, whether it be the heart, the liver, the brain or the chemical interactions therein. If you have an inherited predisposition to disease, this vulnerable part of the body will be the first to be 'conquered' by the stress response.

The stress response may simply be to the ongoing stress of living in the city, to getting married, emigrating or starting a new job – normal life stressors that cannot be avoided easily. They may well be happy stressors, like having a baby, but they are nevertheless stressors that cause this stress-induced hormonal reaction. Again, for the individual who feels as though he or she has always coped well in life, a particular situation suddenly seems insurmountable. It would appear that the individual eventually succeeds, but it's like swimming upstream in order to keep up.

This is a very debilitating experience, equally exhausting to body and mind. It will lead to one or more of the above physical disorders, necessitating consultations with a dietician and psychiatrist. This results in each symptom being examined separately and often treated without achieving the desired results, because both patient and doctor fail to see the 'bigger picture' and find the root cause of the problem. After all, such widespread physical disorders would not automatically lead the sufferer to conclude that the origin is within the brain.

Chronic fatigue syndrome (CFS) and myalgic encephalopathy (ME)

According to much medical literature, CFS and ME are the same syndrome. The symptoms of clinical depression are very similar to those present in CFS and ME. The truth is that all three affect the HPA axis, and they all have overlapping, if not identical, symptoms. The only real difference is that they have differing causes.

Chronic fatigue syndrome is thought to be caused by mononucleosis, or the glandular fever virus, but many other causes are implicated. This virus is able to remain within the host's body after the glandular fever infection has subsided, re-emerging to begin a slow-onset infection when the individual is in a state of compromised immunity (prolonged periods of stress, lack of sleep, or other diseases). Rather than a sudden infection, causing acute and obvious symptoms such as nausea and fever, the virus exerts its effects slowly and discretely. In this way the individual symptoms show themselves, but the virus remains undetected. Testing for the Epstein-Barr virus (EBV) is one way to ascertain whether the person suffers from CFS, although this has recently been questioned. Its presence in the blood will show that this may be a cause of the problem, in which case the best treatment is to treat the symptoms (few viruses respond to antibiotics).

What is sometimes diagnosed as CFS has been treated successfully with anti-depressant drugs. This would lead us to believe that some diagnoses are not chronic fatigue, but actually clinical depression. Does the origin of the illness really matter, if the outcome and the treatment are the same? Remember, though, that together with anti-depressant therapy you require correct nutrition, as well as taking good care of your health to prevent the illness recurring.

The above illustrates the chicken/egg debate. Is there clinical depression latent at the onset of ME or EBV, and the latter simply induced its physical onset? Or, are these infectious diseases that alter the chemicals within the brain responsible for clinical depression? Lastly, could it be that the EBV and ME viruses are not related to clinical depression at all, but simply respond well to the treatment of clinical depression? When it comes to the crunch, does it actually matter? The symptoms are highly debilitating and to me, all seem to come from one disorder with different causes.

DR DORA: People who are perpetually tired: chronic fatigue syndrome

Fatigue is a very common symptom in general practice. In a British study of general practice, 25% of women and 20% of men reported that they feel tired all the time. In other countries too, chronic fatigue is a major problem. About a quarter of Americans attending primary care clinics say constant tiredness is a number one complaint. Is this malaise a symptom of our hectic lifestyle? Not at all. For millennia, physicians have struggled to treat inexplicable fatigue. In the 19th century, the term 'neurasthenia' was coined to describe bodily symptoms such as fatigue, where there was no identifiable *physical* cause. Other favourite names included 'lack of nerve strength'. Sound familiar? Today, we have ME, CFS, yuppie flu and a host of other names.

So, what do patients with CFS have in common? All of them have fatigue that cannot be explained medically. To diagnose it, the fatigue must be spontaneously mentioned by the patient. It also must start suddenly.

Central features of CFS include:

- lack of energy
- weakness
- inability to function – mental fatigue
- flu-like symptoms.

Who gets it?
CFS tends to occur in adults aged 20 to 40 years. It is twice as common in women. Research also shows that men and women describe and explain the illness differently and they are treated differently by the medical profession.[17]

There is much confusion and controversy about CFS. Some people swear it does not exist: it is a 'fad' diagnosis, a basket to catch inexplicable symptoms. Others say it *does* exist but has not been fully understood. To create some order amongst the arguing factions, the Centre for Disease Control (CDC) in the United States has devised specific criteria to make the diagnosis. Even these criteria are controversial! The CDC has identified two major criteria and various symptom criteria that are obtained from the history the patient gives and the physical examination.

The two 'major criteria':
1. There must be a recent onset of persistent or relapsing, debilitating fatigue resulting in at least a 50% reduction in activity, for at least 6 months
2. All other possible diagnoses must be excluded through history, physical examination and laboratory investigations (blood and urine tests).

The physical symptoms are:
1. A mild temperature.
2. Lymph glands are swollen and painful.
3. Unexplained muscle weakness all over the body.
4. Muscles become painful when they are used.
5. For one day after exercise, the sufferer experiences fatigue. This occurs even after a level of exercise that was previously no problem.
6. Headaches occur.
7. Pain flits from joint to joint.
8. From a psychiatric viewpoint, there is memory loss, irritability, poor concentration, depressed mood and sensitivity to light.
9. Sleep disturbance – sleeping too much or too little.
10. The onset must be abrupt.

On physical examination, the doctor finds:
1. A low-grade fever.
2. Signs of an inflamed throat that is not full of pus.
3. Painful swollen lymph nodes in the neck or armpits.

Many people have criticised these criteria as far too complicated. Also, you will notice that all psychiatric patients are excluded. In other words, by definition, a person suffering from depression cannot have the diagnosis of CFS. Is this fair? Many people who develop CFS end up feeling depressed.

CFS is a diagnosis of exclusion. This means that every other medical and psychiatric illness known to cause chronic fatigue must be ruled out.

The million dollar question in CFS is: 'what causes it'? There are many theories and little proof. The list is very long, but the question remains unsolved.

- Infection, with a virus such as Epstein Barr or herpes simplex, is a possibility. But there is so little evidence for the Epstein Barr virus causing CFS that blood tests looking for EBV are no longer recommended. Certain herpes viruses (such as number 6) are also proposed as possible causes, but again, the evidence is weak.

- A compromised immune system may be the culprit. There is some evidence for this, but the findings are inconclusive. People with CFS are more vulnerable to infection and there is some evidence of a compromised stress response.
- Many people have proposed toxins in the diet as the cause. Others point to sugars and yeasts, although again, this rests on flimsy evidence.
- Specific types of neurotransmitters have also been implicated.
- Enzyme problems are a recent theory.[18]

CFS confuses both patients and doctors. It looks very similar to a number of well-described medical illnesses, such as fibromyalgia. This illness is characterised by generalised aches, morning stiffness, muscle pain after exertion. In addition, the sleep quality is poor, with well-described abnormalities on the sleep EEG. It is associated with irritable bowel syndrome, anxiety and depression. On examination, the doctor picks up tender points. Many patients with CFS meet criteria for fibromyalgia. Are they being misdiagnosed?

Another intriguing 'mystery illness' is myalgic encephalitis (ME). Originally ME was called Royal Free Disease, after a hospital in London where an 'epidemic' broke out. It is a puzzling disorder that occurs in small epidemics. It is commoner in women, often those working in institutions (like the original case of the Royal Free Hospital). There are severe symptoms but not much on physical examination. There is no known cause. Most sufferers recover completely. Now, researchers concur that ME and CFS are the same illness.

You may ask, isn't CFS a psychiatric illness? It is true that over two-thirds of patients with a primary complaint of fatigue *are* suffering from a psychiatric condition. Often, these patients have co-existing depression, anxiety, dysthymia and somatisation (where 'emotional' problems are attributed to a physical cause). A family history of depression is extremely common in CFS; in fact as common as in people with major depression.

So, what is the difference between depression and CFS?

- Depressed patients tend to attribute their symptoms to *psychological* factors rather than physical causes
- In depression, guilt and low self-esteem are far more common than in CFS.
- CFS patients generally perform worse on cognitive tests than healthy people, but overall they do better than patients with depression.
- In CFS, memory may be poor – but performance on memory tests fluctuates.
- Depressed people have a loss of confidence about their cognitive decline.
- There are also some differences in the amount of blood flowing through parts of the brain in CFS. These changes in blood flow are not seen in depression.
- Both CFS and depression sufferers have problems with muscle movement, compared with healthy controls.
- But depressed people improve more during the day, especially when it comes to voluntary muscular contraction. CFS sufferers struggle with muscle movement all day long.[19]
  - An intriguing piece of research has examined the responses of 'significant others' to a CFS sufferer. This study tested the effect of a caring response on the *outcome* of CFS. The findings were surprising. Where the significant

other *cared,* the CFS sufferer did *worse.* These caring partners may inadvertently worsen the illness. By helping the patient more with tasks of daily living, they decrease the patient's activity level and independence. This may lead to further disability.[20]

The treatment of CFS is as controversial as the diagnosis. Over 40% of sufferers respond to placebo (an inactive tablet or 'dummy pill'). Lifestyle issues are also important, such as setting limits in work, reducing stress. The role of nutrition is unclear.[21] Certain types of psychotherapy are effective.[22]

Other causes for clinical depression, apart from heredity, are as follows:

- alcohol abuse
- drug abuse
- cortisone therapy (administered for allergies, asthma, in cancer patients, in transplant patients, etc.)
- certain drugs, such as Accutaine® or Roacutane®) (drug prescribed for acne treatment), and some types of oral contraception therapy
- peri- and post-menopause
- anaesthetic (in some people)
- chronic deficiency of pyridoxine (vitamin B6) or metabolic abnormalities concerning pyridoxine
- 'career dieting' (repetitive 'going on diets', or being 'on diet' all the time) – although research is not yet conclusive
- hormonal fluctuations.

DR DORA: What else causes depressed mood?

As we have discussed, genetic factors play an essential role in depression. Against the backdrop of a genetic predisposition or vulnerability, life events and stressors may contribute too. But many other conditions may mimic depression.

- Depression occurs in many neurological illnesses, such as Alzheimer's dementia, Parkinson's disease, stroke, syphilis and epilepsy.
- Infections are another cause of depression: HIV, TB and pneumonia are all culprits.
- Inflammatory conditions of the joints and connective tissue (rheumatoid arthritis, for example) cause depression.
- Many tumours present with depression *first.*

It doesn't stop here – over 100 medications that are used routinely can cause depression, including:

- anti-hypertensives
- appetite suppressants
- antibiotics
- anti-fungals
- anti-cancer drugs
- pain killers
- oral contraceptives.

Again, if the individual is genetically predisposed to clinical depression, these factors may be triggers to the onset of clinical depression. So, if you have had any of the alternative treatments or have abused drugs or alcohol and have noticed a slow but dramatic negative change in your psychiatric well-being, you should consider professional assessment. Don't wait until this condition ruins your life, relationships, work and self-esteem. The psychological setbacks created in this way will simply add to the psychiatric recovery time.

Remember that there is nothing to be ashamed of. There is often nothing wrong with your psychological make up – yet! So, go for a check-up, just like you would have your eyes or your thyroid tested. The worst that can happen (or the best!) is that the psychiatrist tells you that you have nothing to worry about at all, and sends you home with a clean bill of mental health!

Often symptoms of a 'latent' clinical depression are evident in childhood, if there is ADHD (attention deficit hyperactivity disorder) or separation anxiety displayed in the child. The increased level of anxiety seen in some children may in fact be a small indication of clinical depression which may exacerbate itself in later life.

Although clinical depression is a chronic and debilitating disorder (even fatal), treatment is now so advanced that a relatively quick recovery can be made under correct psychiatric supervision. If you suffer from clinical depression you will not automatically be admitted to a psychiatric ward – only if you fail to treat the disease and become suicidal. For the average clinical depression sufferer, a few visits to the psychiatrist will do the trick in determining the type of treatment that is needed, and ensuring its efficacy.

But let's talk about diet, now.

5 CARBOHYDRATES AND SEROTONIN

Having examined the activities of the hypothalamus and how it relates to the rest of the body, it should be clear why clinical depression is almost identical to persistent anxiety, and how incorrect serotonin function results in both conditions. Moreover, clinical depression is not a disorder of the brain alone; it affects the rest of your body as well.

To treat clinical depression you have to consult a medical professional, and probably take some medication. Furthermore, changing your life and mindset will empower you to prevent depression re-occurring. Then there is the nutrition link. As a dietician, my knowledge of nutrition provides the background for this book. Read on and discover for yourself how the function of serotonin is linked to carbohydrates.

I think that by now you will have understood why I had to go to such lengths in order to explain how non-threatening clinical depression and the prescribed treatment with antidepressants really are. So, I hope that those clinical depressives out there have made an appointment to see a psychiatrist, or have explained to a friend or relative how she can start getting better.

Women and depression

As explained in chapter 2, more women are documented as suffering from clinical depression than men, but that does not preclude men from suffering from the condition. Women often find it easier to talk about themselves and their problems than men; yet many men are diagnosed with clinical depression. So chaps, read along too, you may learn a lot!

The following section will apply to practically all women, and many, many men (even if it is just empathetic reading to better understand their partners!). Every woman I have ever met has wanted to know more about the link between food and depression and I have come to the conclusion that the 'food' issue applies to nearly every single woman on earth, but not necessarily to all men. By the end of this chapter you will understand exactly why there is a link between food and depression – and it has a lot to do with hormones.

Serotonin

As the previous chapters described, serotonin is produced to deliver the response of 'calm'. Serotonin does not sedate. If you need to be alert to act in a panic situation serotonin does not prevent alertness. It merely 'controls' the response. Neither does it make you happy. With plenty of serotonin present, you feel good and content, but if something occurs that makes you unhappy, serotonin cannot prevent that effect. However, it does help you to cope better under the circumstances. So, it is not an override button for happiness either.

A good way to describe what serotonin does it is to say that it holds the potential for a sense of positive well-being. Other than that, it tempers and organises the other brain chemicals to work efficiently. Besides your mood and psychological make-up, others factors also affect the production of serotonin. Two of these are oestrogen and blood sugar levels.

Oestrogen

This obviously applies to female readers, but men, please read and learn. Many of you could do with a crash course in female biology. Oestrogen is a wonderful female sex hormone that provides women with beautiful breasts, curvy waists and hips and voluptuous thighs, among other things. Because oestrogen is also the primary hormone that prepares a woman's body for the conception of a baby and the subsequent pregnancy, its concentration in the blood increases and decreases by the day. Each month, the body is again ready for pregnancy, and the woman can do nothing but allow these hormones to hold their sway while trying to live a normal life, continue with her job, be a gorgeous and loving wife, and an ever-caring and giving mother, whilst riding on the emotional roller-coaster of hormonal fluctuations.

The menstrual cycle starts on the first day of bleeding. From this day, the hormone levels (oestrogen and progesterone) start rising, increasing daily, in preparation for conception. An egg is released from the ovary in the middle of the month. If this egg is fertilised, the hormone levels simply continue to increase, thickening the uterus lining to accommodate the growing baby. Only once the baby has been born do the hormones return to normal levels.

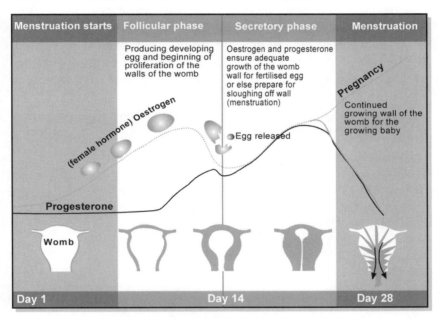

However, if the egg is not fertilised, oestrogen and progesterone start decreasing (they are not needed), and then suddenly plummet to baseline in order to let the body know that the uterus lining needs to be expelled (a period). Once the bleeding commences, so does the next menstrual cycle and the oestrogen levels increase again. This cycle is usually 28-31 days.

Oestrogen is a very powerful hormone that has widespread effects on nearly every part of a woman's body. No wonder women feel different from one day to the next! Most (though not all) women feel especially appalling just before they menstruate. This is called premenstrual syndrome (PMS) and symptoms include the following:

- irritability
- tearfulness
- poor memory
- poor concentration

- lack of energy
- changes in appetite
- changes in weight
- water retention
- lethargy
- sleep disturbances
- headaches and migraines.

If you have been reading this book carefully, you will know exactly what these are: symptoms of acute (quick-onset) clinical depression! Fortunately, PMS lasts only a couple of days and requires patience and TLC, no medication. As oestrogen levels increase or decrease, so serotonin production changes accordingly.

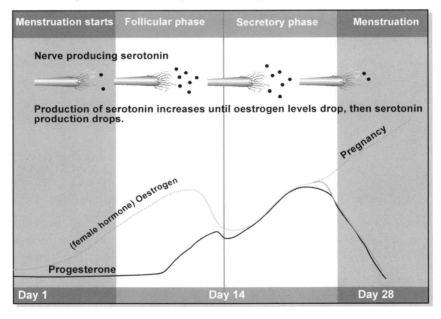

Serotonin function also changes with the post-partum plummet in oestrogen levels. During pregnancy the oestrogen level increases over the nine-month period, until suddenly it drops, for the birth. In someone who is prone to developing clinical depression or persistent anxiety, this is often when medication is needed – especially since this kind of hypothalamic disruption will inhibit prolactin (for breastfeeding).

Getting back to the monthly hormones. Women are usually fine until the 5-10 days before menstruation. Then hormones turn them into impatient, irrational, tearful and horribly bloated monsters.

The craving for sugar is not only emotional, it is powerfully hormonal in its origin, too.

The oestrogen content in the blood influences serotonin production. So when oestrogen production drops, so does serotonin production. In clinical depressives, barely any of this serotonin reaches the hypothalamus anyway, but it is certainly being helped by oestrogen-stimulated increases in serotonin production. Then oestrogen decreases and serotonin effects fade into oblivion ...

The anxiety and clinical depression will remain until such time as the body's oestrogen levels increase and the hypothalamus can start behaving normally again (or at least as normally as the reuptake site will allow). Until that time, the body feels at a loss, and naturally looks for other things to compensate for that mood. One of these compensatory mechanisms is sugar.

Sugar?

Yes, sugar! If the blood sugar level increases, so does serotonin production, and voilà! A better balance of chemicals again, but only for a while ... We are about to explore that in detail, but first, just be aware that your cravings for 'simple' carbohydrates (as they used to be called) are there for a very good reason, and denying yourself the pleasure of them may not be the best thing at all.

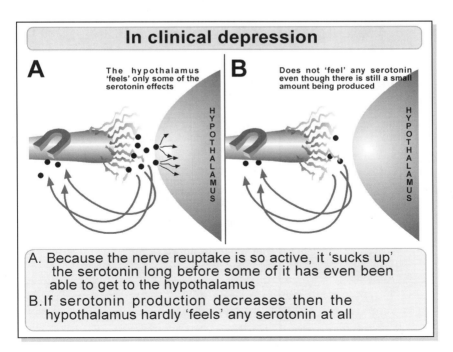

In clinical depression

A The hypothalamus 'feels' only some of the serotonin effects

B Does not 'feel' any serotonin even though there is still a small amount being produced

A. Because the nerve reuptake is so active, it 'sucks up' the serotonin long before some of it has even been able to get to the hypothalamus

B. If serotonin production decreases then the hypothalamus hardly 'feels' any serotonin at all

We are going to get a little technical here. All you have to do is to understand and keep remembering that the depressive only 'feels' the effects of a small amount of the serotonin that is being produced, and so when serotonin production decreases, the depressive 'feels' nearly no serotonin at all.

When serotonin production increases, the depressive doesn't experience the increase as an overwhelming sense of well-being (like most people do). This individual only 'feels' the effect of some of the serotonin. This increase in serotonin makes the 'serotonin-deaf' depressive feel almost 'normal', like all other healthy people feel daily. It is only natural that the depressive would try to achieve this feeling as often as possible. One way to succeed is to instinctively 'self-medicate' with sugars which stimulate more serotonin production.

Serotonin is a chemical manufactured inside the serotonin-producing nerve, from an amino acid called tryptophan, crucial to the manufacture of serotonin. The amount of tryptophan received into the nerve determines how much serotonin can be made. But the amount of tryptophan that enters the nerve depends on other amino acids in the blood as well.

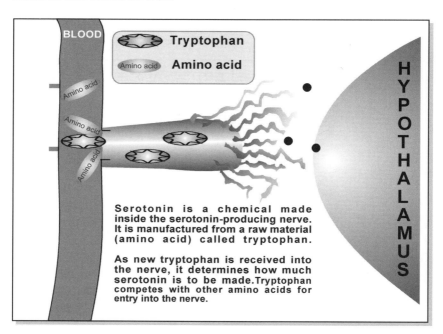

The opening where tryptophan enters the nerve from the blood is the same opening through which all amino acids enter from the blood, resulting in the amino acids competing for entry. Tryptophan is the least likely of all the amino acids to successfully enter the opening. Think of it as the 'runt of the litter'. When there are lots of other amino acids in the blood, like after a light protein meal, less tryptophan will be able to enter the nerve, and in turn, less serotonin will be produced. If, however, there are less amino acids in the blood, then tryptophan can enter the nerve with greater ease, ready to form serotonin.

But how can the amino acid concentration in the blood be decreased? With insulin!

The main function of insulin is to store! If there is a lot of insulin present in the blood, it will store the amino acids into the muscles. Insulin therefore lowers the concentration of amino acids in the blood, affording tryptophan greater opportunity to enter the nerve and form serotonin. And insulin is produced in response to carbohydrates!

When you eat carbohydrates, they dissolve into component sugars that fill the blood. This high sugar level stimulates the 'storage police' (insulin) to come out and move the sugar into the muscles where it is needed for energy. But, while the insulin stores sugar from the blood into the muscles, it is also storing amino acids into the muscles, leaving the tryptophan free to enter the nerve. So, indirectly, carbohydrates contribute to a physiological improvement in psychological well-being.

Do all carbohydrates do this? Yes! Some more than others, however, depending on how quickly these carbohydrates dissolve into sugars ... in other words, according to the glycaemic index of each carbohydrate.

All carbohydrates consist of sugar. When you eat any carbohydrate, it dissolves into sugar in the blood. Some carbohydrates, such as bread, potatoes and maize meal, are made up of sugar which is held together by very loose bonds. When eaten, they dissolve into sugar very quickly. We call them high glycaemic index carbohydrates, with a GI of 100 (all GI counts are numbers out of 100), and so this is the highest, or fastest-dissolving carbohydrate.

Other carbohydrates, such as sweet potatoes, basmati rice and pearled barley ('gort') are also made up of sugar, but the sugar molecules are held together by very strong bonds. Because they are held together very tightly, they take much longer to dissolve into the blood. As such, we call them low GI carbohydrates, and they have a GI ranging from 40-21.

So, when you eat high GI carbohydrates, large amounts of insulin are produced to store the sugar and the amino acids, thus allowing more tryptophan into the nerve, to produce serotonin. Now that you understand exactly how this all occurs, it would suffice to say, albeit simplistically, that high GI carbohydrates cause more serotonin to be produced in the brain.

GLYCAEMIC INDEX EXCHANGE

Carbohydrate	GI
Cornflakes/ Rice Crispies/ Mealie meal	100
White/ Brown/ Wholewheat/ French bread	100
Honey	100
Puffed Wheat	100
Weet Bix	100
Potato – mashed	100
Potato – baked	100
Crispbread	89
Rye bread	89
Instant rice	87
Rice cakes	81
Potato – boiled	80
Coco Pops/ Frosties	77
Bagel	72
Gnocchi	68
Oatso Easy ·	66
Brown rice	66
Peas, green	65
Cous cous	61
Sweet corn (plain or creamed)	60
Baked beans	60
Ryvita/ Finn Crisp	59
Cane sugar	59
Basmati rice	58
Haricot beans	57
All Bran flakes/ Special K	54
White rice – parboiled	54
Oats porridge	47
Potato, Sweet	46
Butter beans	46
Chick peas	40
Pasta (all types, cooked al dente)	40
Lentils	28
Fructose	22
Pearled barley	22
Soy beans/ soy mince	21

Taken from *The GI Factor,* by Dr J Brand Miller.

And you thought that it was just you who thought that a slice of bread and jam made you feel better! Well, honey, it makes everyone feel better! Especially if they are feeling down in the dumps.

Not only do high GI carbohydrates (indirectly) stimulate serotonin production in a big way, they also stimulate the production to take place very quickly! When you feel down, anxious, or just downright lonely, it is no coincidence that you subconsciously 'self-medicate' by craving high GI foods, such as bread, sweets, maize meal, popcorn, cola, mashed or baked potatoes, cakes and crisps. These are all quick-fix serotonin boosters! And yes, they do make you feel better. That is why it isn't merely a matter of your body wanting these foods, it really needs to have them.

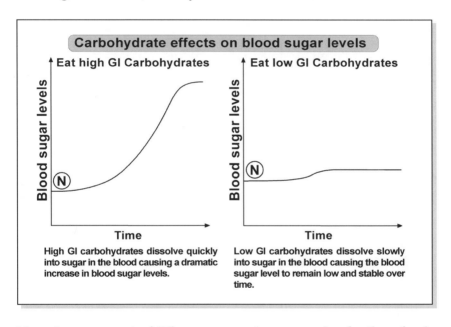

Carbohydrate effects on blood sugar levels

Eat high GI Carbohydrates

Eat low GI Carbohydrates

High GI carbohydrates dissolve quickly into sugar in the blood causing a dramatic increase in blood sugar levels.

Low GI carbohydrates dissolve slowly into sugar in the blood causing the blood sugar level to remain low and stable over time.

Never ignore a craving! When you experience a craving for these foods this is your body's way of signalling that it needs something to correct what has gone wrong. Satisfy the craving first, then ascertain its cause. Either your sugar levels are too low or you may be feeling depressed. Perhaps your life is filled with anxiety. Maybe you are pre-menstrual. Perhaps you are suffering from a psychiatric disorder, such as clinical depression. Deal with the root cause of the craving in whatever way is required. You may require professional help, either from your family doctor, or from a psychologist or psychiatrist. Either way, take time out to assess your life and search for the reasons for your behaviour.

DR DORA: Tryptophan

It has been known for some time that when *certain* carbohydrates are eaten, the serotonin precursor, tryptophan, becomes more readily available to the brain.[1] Hence more serotonin can be produced. This premise was tested when women with premenstrual tension participated in a four-month study.[2] During the trial they received three carbohydrate-rich drinks: two that did not affect serotonin production at all and one concoction that was known to increase tryptophan levels. Mood, intellectual ability and food cravings were tested before and after they had the drink. Only the tryptophan-promoting drink significantly decreased depression, anger, confusion and carbohydrate craving in these women – possibly because serotonin levels were enhanced.

Whether or not it is one of the above, craving something rather than just wanting it means that you probably aren't getting enough serotonin activity. So, if listening to your body and eating high GI carbohydrates is such an obvious route to alleviate the problem, why have we always been told this is wrong?

- The myth still prevails that carbohydrates make us fat, which is untrue.
- We are ignorant about how much fat is actually hidden in many of these foods, posing dangers to our weight and health.
- Often in anxiety-prone individuals, eating only high GI carbohydrates can cause a consequent dip in blood sugar levels which is unhealthy. Also, using just high GI carbohydrates to elevate moods can be dangerous for insulin-resistant individuals and diabetics.
- We are only just beginning to understand how to use carbohydrates to our advantage, using the Glycaemic Index. But more of that later...

Before having fun with carbohydrates please read to the end of this book to understand the complexities of GI manipulation. It is ignorance surrounding carbohydrates which has led many of us to see food as the enemy.

6 WHY IS FOOD THE ENEMY?

When I read a women's magazine featuring yet another article on the latest four-day weight-loss plan, I become truly bitter with anger. When will this insanity stop? Quick weight-loss programmes and tasteless starvation regimes are as harmful to your body and mind as they are impossible to maintain.

I have had a bellyful of this perpetual half-cocked and dangerous knowledge that wrecks lives, and I would like to share my knowledge so that we can respect our bodies and treat them the way they deserve – with honour. Fat loss and dieting are DIFFICULT, but can be managed successfully once one is treading an informed path.

DR DORA: Fad diets come and go, but the extra weight stays and grows...

This is the conclusion after several decades of 'quick fix' solutions. From a medical point of view, there is no evidence that these fashionable diets work.

- 'Mono-nutrient diets' that severely restrict food intake to one source (grapes, rice, you name it) are dangerous. They supposedly 'cleanse' the body – of what? There is no scientific evidence that any cleansing occurs. In the long run, they deprive the body of a variety of nutrients and may cause malnutrition.

- 'Crash diets' sweepingly restrict food intake. Initially, they tend to result in water loss; then muscle tissue goes. Fat stores go last. It is impossible to maintain such a diet. With the body in a state of semi-starvation, food craving is inevitable and the weight loss is steadily regained, often more than before the diet started (see *The X Diet* for more information).

- The benefits of 'food-combining diets' (where proteins and carbohydrates are not eaten together) have not been proven effective in the scientific literature. If any weight loss does occur, it is believed to be the result of eating *less overall*. Preparing food becomes too much bother because separating protein from the starch is so complicated. Meals tend to lack in overall nutrition or are simply skipped. A recent study[1] examined the effect of a normal balanced diet versus a food-combined diet in obese people. There was no difference in the amount of weight loss or fat loss in the two groups!

The functioning of a healthy brain relies on a steady supply of nutrients, water and oxygen. Talk about a refined diet – the brain depends on *blood glucose* to fuel most of what it does in keeping us alive. The brain is our most vital and sensitive organ, so we have evolved to protect it from the chaos that might be raging in other parts of the body or bloodstream. The 'blood-brain barrier' is the 'border control' that prevents other nutrients, like fats and large proteins, from reaching the brain. Wreaking havoc with one's blood sugar levels through crash dieting may lead to serious problems because the brain cannot rely on other food sources for energy.

A study examining the mental performance of dieters found that they tend to do worse on tests of concentration and memory compared to non-dieters.[2]

Sorely restricting protein intake starves the brain in a different way. Essential protein building blocks called *amino acids* can penetrate the blood-brain barrier to enter brain tissue. Here they are modified into the chemical messengers the brain uses to communicate (neurotransmitters). Many of these amino acids can only be obtained from food: they cannot be manufactured in the brain. Cutting out protein may lead to low levels of essential amino acids, resulting in correspondingly low levels of neurotransmitters. Without these chemical messengers, brain cells struggle to communicate with each other. Interfering with the brain's communication network leads to a host of psychiatric and physical problems.

The fact that many medical aids do not cover dietetically controlled weight control programmes proves that our society still regards them as an unnecessary and vain affliction. If you could join me in the clinic for one day you would have first-hand knowledge of the serious nature of obesity, and gain insight into how widespread the associated disease of depression really is. You too will leave with a feeling of despair and anger at the misinformation created by the ignorant, and share my zeal for education to prevent more people from being sucked into a spiral of panic, fear and hopelessness.

Strong words indeed, but read on. Once you have learnt the truth about dieting and depression, you will never diet again. You will probably be as indignant as many of my patients who constantly ask: 'Why isn't this information known? Why is no one ever told this? It seems as though this information is being hidden from us!'

DR DORA: What is obesity?

Obesity is the excessive accumulation of body fat. Traditionally, standardised height-weight tables were used to calculate ideal weight. If one weighed over 20% more than that expected for one's height, one was considered obese. An increasingly popular way of determining nutritional status is with 'body mass index'. This requires some arithmetic! Mass in kilograms is divided by height in metres squared. (Mass/Height^2). If the result obtained is over 30, the person is classified obese; if between 25 and 30, overweight. Despite all the solid scientific evidence of the dangers of obesity, the incidence of obesity is rising in the developed world. For example, more than half of American adults are overweight or obese.[3] Over one quarter of North American adults are classified obese (24% of men and 27% of women). Similar rates are true for Europe. If this trend continues, in 20 years' time many more will be overweight.[4]

Obesity is a disease

Firstly, this information is not being hidden from us – the medical profession simply does not acknowledge the need to continuously update research on weight loss. A great part of this profession still holds the view that obesity is a result of laziness and gluttony, and that there is only one way to get thin: Eat less, and you'll be fine!

THIS IS WRONG! Obesity is a deadly disease and its treatment is of global concern. It is also difficult to cure and requires specialised treatment, often involving more than one therapy. Obesity can cause many, if not most, lifestyle disorders that people suffer from. Here are but a few:

- cancer
- diabetes
- cholesterol problems
- blood pressure problems
- irregular periods and infertility
- polycystic ovarian syndrome
- kidney disease
- inflammatory disease, such as arthritis and gout
- depression and low self-esteem
- lower back pain
- arthritis of the knees and ankles
- skin problems
- lowered work productivity
- broken marriages (You have no idea how prevalent this is – not because of obesity itself, but as a result of the trauma associated with constant dieting and the concurrent financial costs of dieting!)

- other psychiatric disorders
- psychological damage
- ongoing infections and ill health.

DR DORA: More on the medical complications of obesity

Obesity is associated with increased illness and earlier death.[5] But it is not as simple as more fat equals more risk. Precisely *where* fat is distributed on your body has been shown to affect vulnerability to various illnesses. Excess fat around the abdomen or trunk is associated with an increased risk of coronary artery disease and even early death. If the blood vessels bringing blood to the heart muscle (coronary arteries) become blocked, the heart tissue starves and dies. This is initially experienced as chest pain, and later as heart attacks.

Where there is excessive fat around the hips and thighs (more common in women), there does not appear to be the same cardiac risk.

However, obese women suffer their own particular risks. Being obese and pregnant is a very bad combination. There is increased risk for high blood pressure and diabetes during the pregnancy as well as maternal and foetal mortality. Overweight women are more likely to have Caesarean deliveries. Unfortunately, surgical complications frequently arise. Babies born to obese mothers are often blue at birth, may have spinal cord abnormalities and are more likely to die in the weeks following birth.[6]

A fascinating recent research finding is that the bodily distribution of fat changes in depressed people; even in those people who lose their appetites. In depression, fat stores tend to *redistribute* around their abdomens. If the depression is untreated, they may suffer from the associated risks of truncal obesity. This may be caused by high levels of the stress hormone, cortisol, in depression.

For obvious health reasons there is great pressure on the obese to be slim. There is also sustained pressure from society, linking success with a slim figure in the workplace, in social situations, in romantic relationships, etc. This continuous pressure, not only on the obese, but on all women, creates unrealistic expectations that often cannot be met.

'Nice and thin'

A paediatric endocrinologist referred Jessie (name changed), a little girl of nine to the clinic. She suffered from a variety of problems (and she was not even fat). She carried a little extra 'puppy fat', but the impact it had on her young life was nothing short of petrifying.

Though she is highly intelligent, her performance at school suffered, her friends shunned her and she became withdrawn.

I spent weeks talking to her, and consulted with her school and her mother to establish the root of her problem. Eventually she confessed to her mother that she 'wasn't a nice person'. Shocked, her mother asked why would she think that. She answered, very matter-of-factly, 'Well, all the girls at school know that I am not a nice girl.'

Confused, her mother asked why she would think so. Did she tell lies? Did she hit the other girls? Did she take things from them? Did she play rough? (All these things did not fit her character at all.)

Her reason was quite simple: All her friends' mothers spoke of being 'nice and thin', and because Jessie was not thin, her friends saw her quite simply as 'not nice' and therefore wouldn't play with her. This is a completely true story.

What on earth are we doing? This ostensibly harmless phrase, 'nice and thin', becomes an opinion that filters through to a generation of youngsters who are pressured enough as it is, and sets a new expectation – one that most might never reach. The resultant poor self-esteem speaks for itself.

What is sexy?

Instead of publicising these horror stories and making known the dangers of fat-fears, society will keep ploughing out more and more anorexic success stories: the beautiful supermodel Kate Moss; the successful Ally McBeal, a character in the TV series by the same name; and the Oscar award-winning actress Gwyneth Paltrow. None of these women succeeds in conveying a picture of health or femininity. They are painfully thin and appear frail to the point of looking ill.

Femininity used to be associated with softness, curves, dimpled smiles and voluptuous breasts. Marilyn Monroe is a good example of such femininity.

Now there seems to be a warped attitude that the successful female should have the body of a thirteen-year-old boy – a flat-chested, bony fragility of 'not quite being there'. Apparently we are ashamed of our womanhood and sexuality; so ashamed that we aspire to achieve a body clearly incapable of reproduction. Why are we ashamed of oestrogen, the very hormone that sets us apart from men?

No wonder this global panic has given food the shocking name it has. After all, someone who is able to resist the never-ending appeal of food gets thin, and thin is nice. Too often we hear: 'thin is successful', or 'you can never be too rich or too thin'.

On the other hand, we often envy relationships in which the

feminine half laughs with sexy abandon and drizzles honey onto her toast in a way that leaves most men breathless. Lovely Kathleen Turner was once called someone who very obviously 'loves the feeling of a sundress moving over her soft skin'. How delicious to be someone who simply enjoys what her body feels like! The secret of her success (and of those other less 'physically successful' women whose relationships turn us green with envy), is that there is no secret. There is simply nothing to hide!

These women are proud to look different from their 13-year-old brothers. They are proud to show their curves, and delight in moving and sitting in ways that attract attention to their femininity.

They are successful because they accept what they are: feminine! They love being women, and their partners love that confidence, that sense of sexy abandon that these women seem to carry with them.

Continental women demonstrate this quality well. Any French beach packed with topless female sunbathers will reveal that very few Frenchwomen have succumbed to plastic surgery. They proudly display their different shapes and sizes. This confidence in their own femininity instantly transforms these ordinary and differently shaped women into sex symbols. They are able to forget about their bodies, and concentrate on being fun to be with, cheeky, content and, above all, flirtatious.

We are all happy to say that we like being brunettes, blondes or redheads. We appreciate that men are attracted to these individual aspects of us. But why can't we appreciate our unique and individual shapes and allow ourselves to show them off? Could it be because women have entrenched the idea that a man is only successful if he is with a 'successful' and thin wife, ('nice and thin')? Meanwhile men enjoy looking at voluptuous girls in magazines, the epitome of curvaceous femininity!

Let's stop worrying about the negative aspects of our bodies and rather focus on our strengths. This way we can truly appreciate the things that matter – such as the sensory pleasure of feeling how your body moves seductively to the beat of music; how perfume warms in the nape of your neck; the beautiful curve of your bottom and the small of your back, and the soft smoothness of your thigh.

With this apparent quest for zero defect, we as women are allowing ourselves to move from 'penis envy' to 'complete man envy', wanting to look as rock-hard, unshapely and muscularly defined as possible. Are these not qualities of the male body? And aren't the differences that our hormones bless us with the very essence of feminine power and attraction?

May I mention how seductive food can be? Compare the impact of the movies '9 ½ Weeks', or 'When Harry met Sally' to marry the perception of food and sexuality once and for all.

DR DORA: When did the quest for thinness start?

Many people believe that anorexia nervosa is an illness of modern times, when one can never be 'too rich or too thin'. The anorexic's skeletal face is considered the *extreme* of the modern quest for ultimate thinness. Down the line, anorexics look shocking, rather than desirable. But still they refuse food. They seem to have lost sight of how unappealing they have become. If one studies the medical literature, one discovers that this behaviour is not new. Anorexia nervosa was given its medical name and description in the second half of the 19th century but voluntary starvation has been around for much longer.[7] Since ancient times, there have been reports of various eating disorders. From generation to generation, these have differed in their frequency and the way they present clinically. The standards for feminine beauty change over the decades and along with them, the common eating disorders change too.[8]

Why is food the enemy?

Let's return to the burning issue: why food is our enemy. A woman's need for food transcends natural appetite and follows her hormonal changes. But we also strive for the apparently unattainable goal of a 'successful', gauntly thin body. The constant struggle between what our bodies require and giving in to the pressure of society to stay slim, leads us to view food as the natural enemy. Our innate desire for food burdens us constantly with guilt and keeps us from achieving true success and happiness.

DR DORA: Moods, food and the menstrual cycle

Premenstrually, millions of women experience irritability, minor mood swings and a host of other symptoms. Only in a minority of women, premenstrual tension is an incapacitating condition that seriously disrupts their lives. These women may experience markedly depressed mood, anxiety, an inability to concentrate, fatigue, anger and some physical symptoms such as breast tenderness. The prevalence rate in the community has been estimated in various studies to be between 3% and 9% of women.[9-13] The DSM IV term for this condition is a mouthful: premenstrual dysphoric disorder (PMDD). In psychiatric jargon, dysphoria means low mood. There are many theories about why certain women develop this serious condition. In addition to hormonal changes, a variety of neurotransmitters – including serotonin – have been implicated.

Eating patterns definitely change during the menstrual cycle. In PMDD, the DSM IV specifies that there is either marked change in appetite, overeating or specific food desires.[14] Most commonly, carbohydrates (starchy and sugary foods) are craved. Believe it or not, there is a biological reason for this quirky behaviour. Only recently have researchers understood why premenstrual women crave carbohydrate-rich foods. These women may be attempting to increase serotonin levels in their brains. It has been known for some time that when *certain* carbohydrates are eaten, the serotonin precursor, tryptophan, becomes more readily available to the brain.[15] This means that more serotonin can be produced.

Women with premenstrual tension participated in a four-month study that examined carbohydrate cravings during the menstrual cycle.[16] During the trial they received three carbohydrate-rich drinks: two that did not affect serotonin production at all and one concoction that was known to increase tryptophan levels. Mood, intellectual ability and food cravings were tested before and after they had the drink. Only the tryptophan-promoting drink significantly decreased depression, anger, confusion and carbohydrate craving in these women – possibly because serotonin levels were enhanced. So, it's no mystery why grumpy premenstrual women crave sweet things – they are self-medicating by increasing their serotonin levels!

There are many other nutritional theories related to PMDD. For example, both calcium and vitamin D have been implicated. We know that ovarian hormones influence the metabolism of calcium, magnesium and vitamin D. It has been known for many years that decreased calcium levels cause mood disorders – and these closely resemble the low mood of PMDD. Calcium supplementation may treat PMDD symptoms.[17]

Can you see what I'm getting at? We must produce good food. We must eat good food, and we must savour and appreciate its pleasures. We must enjoy food the way it is meant to be enjoyed.

The more we deny our appetites, the stronger becomes the attraction to food. And I don't only mean psychologically, either. The obsession with food is not only psychologically driven, but is hormonally and physiologically based, too. A hard case to contest when you finally understand it.

This attitude of 'Food is the enemy and you are its victim' shows a blatant ignorance of basic physiology. It is perpetuated by the fact that some people still view weight control as a see-saw formula. (The difference between how many calories you eat and how many you burn must result in a body change, whether gaining or losing weight.) Come on guys! The medical fraternity has known since the sixties that calories all behave differently, and that a simple calorie imbalance does not cause obesity.

Doctors and dieting

Are some practitioners really so hungry for wealth that they completely forget what they have learnt about nutrition and surge ahead with severe calorie-cutting and quick fixes? Are they really so result-driven as not to consider what damage they are causing to their patients? Is it really too much of an effort to acknowledge the dangers of calorie-cutting, and try to protect people from damage?

Maybe. After all, the drive towards thinness has created an insatiable financial demand for body-shrinking, whatever the cost! Why worry about medical ethics that protect the patient, when the lucrative little slimming business set up under the auspices of the ever-respected white coat provides such good income? 'He's a doctor, after all,' we murmur respectfully, 'and he says he has specialised in weight control and nutrition.'

Why, then, won't some doctors reveal what they are injecting into their patients? Why do they allow you to experience hunger pains, emotional anxiety and feelings of guilt when you 'succumb' to your body's natural survival signal – hunger?

Something is amiss here, and I think we should all catch a wake-up call.

I do not wish to slate the entire medical fraternity. I refer to those doctors who set themselves up as weight loss specialists, instead of practising as the GPs or gynaecologists they are. They practise outside of their field of expertise, knowing little more about dietetics than the basic Starvation Principle. These doctors promote restrictive diets and appetite suppressants that are addictive and cause psychological problems. They conveniently discard the ever-increasing evidence that this form of starvation slimming may be effective in the short term, but extremely dangerous in the long term. Their ultimate goal is to get the patient to slim down rapidly, whilst giving the impression that they are acting in the patient's best interest.

Perhaps their motives are benevolent, but look at the patient after the drastic slimming. She may not have obesity-related disorders, but, wow look at her now! Clinical depression, lethargy, food obsessions, social maladjustment and infertility to boot! Curing the disease of obesity with blatant disregard for what the methods may be doing to the patient's health is shocking, to say the least.

Having said this, I would like to reiterate that I am only against those doctors who practise unethical methods in slimming; who claim to be what they are not (in other words, they are not clinical dieticians). I remain a proud member of mainstream medicine.

In fact, the huge swing away from conventional medicine to alternative healing is precisely the black-and-white naïveté I am so opposed to. Patients who think that I can heal cancer with diet and herbs get an earful from me. We cannot possibly do away with doctors and medicine!

Instead we should move with the times and identify what mistakes the medical fraternity has made in the field of weight loss, banish those dangerous ideas and move forward with medical research to create new weight loss programmes that won't harm the patient. The medical fraternity provides an irreplaceable and vital service, and this we must respect. Likewise, professionals must respect each other's different fields of expertise.

'You are what you eat'

The old adage 'you are what you eat' refers to the kinds of molecules (i.e. nutrients) that enter your body in the form of food and how they benefit your health. It does not refer to how much you eat. If these nutrients are absent in the body it leads to deficiency diseases. This is often a result of diet regimens that work for weight loss, but cause deficiencies which give rise to headaches, ulcers, cold sores, depression, lethargy, etc.

So people get fat because they have eaten too much, right? Wrong! (Read **The X Diet** to understand just how wrong that is.) Nevertheless, the opinion is still held very firmly. After all, 'Just look at how much that fat person eats!' If, on the other hand, a slim person ate a lot, you would probably envy her quietly rather than think ill of it. Believe me, it's not how much a person eats, it's what she eats, as well as the other aspects of her life asserting powerful yet ignored effects on her body. Simply thinking that someone eats too much is far too simplistic. In reality it is far more complex than such simple observational 'logic': very much like watching my husband settling down to watch cricket! It takes between one and two hours for him to doze off. Can I therefore conclude that cricket is an effective replacement for sleeping pills, and that insomniacs should watch cricket in their bedrooms? Of course not! You cannot draw a conclusion based on what looks obvious.

Fat is fattening

Eating too much fat for the amount of exercise that you do will make you fat, especially if you have a weight problem, like suffering from Syndrome X (See Chapter 1 in **The X Diet**). If you cut out fat, and eat as much of everything else you like, you will not get fat. It's that simple. But this only emerged with research. Prior popular opinion held that sugary foods are fattening, as are tasty foods. They should therefore be avoided at all costs.

When you watch an overweight person eating a huge slice of cake you naturally (or conveniently) assume that the cake is fattening because

1. it is sweet, so sugar must be fattening,
2. it tastes good, so anything tasty must be fattening.

But you forget that besides sugar, cake is also made with butter.

This may sound silly, but historically we have accepted that sugar is fattening and that tasty foods are bad for us. Many of us have subjected ourselves to tasteless and dangerous weight-loss programmes based on these fallacies. The hapless inmates of concentration camps got thin because they had nothing to eat. To earn a fast buck, some medical practitioners and diet clubs prescribe the same type of starvation diet – but under a different name!

The 'perfect diet' for weight loss

Pardon my sarcasm, but using these deductions, I have formulated the 'perfect' weight-loss diet:

1. Make sure the diet is tasteless.
2. Make sure it resembles anything but the traditional foods we have always celebrated, such as those eaten at Christmas, weddings, batmitzvahs or romantic dinners.
3. Ensure that the diet plan is completely different from what the rest of your family eats. This will make you feel perpetually deprived and miserable, and you will have to spend twice as long in the kitchen to prepare two separate menus – one for the family and one for you.
4. Banish all thoughts of culinary pleasure – to enjoy food means to get fat; to hate your food guarantees a figure like that of Kate Moss.
5. Do whatever you can to avoid eating:
   - Take pills that induce the shakes and palpitations.

- Stick a photo of the 'fat you' on the fridge as a perpetual reminder of your failures; forcing you to continue to starve.
- Hire someone else to do the cooking (even if you can't afford it) just so that you are not tempted.
- Buy a portable scale so that you can learn to ignore your natural needs and follow those of a hypothetical body that does not exist.

6. Step on the bathroom scale at least twice a day. After all, the scale never lies, does it? Even if you are premenstrual, constipated, have just eaten a meal, and drunk three litres of water – if the scale has gone up, it cannot possibly be anything else besides an out-of-control, obese body. Then make sure you chastise yourself at least five times every hour.

7. If you view food as anything other than an evil addiction, eat less. The realisation that all food is evil will find you. It finds everyone.

8. Always remember that food will never be your friend. The rewarding feelings you get from food are for people who deserve it. Not you! You are a failure. You don't deserve food. Hasn't anyone told you?

9. If you show any signs of human weakness (such as a chocolate every now and then), prepare yourself for the consequences. You are a naughty girl who needs constant reminding not to be bad. And remember, you are the only one who has ever bent the rules. So when you go for the weekly weigh-in, you deserve to sit with the 'failures' and feel thoroughly useless and weak-willed: a complete glutton with no self-respect at all, in fact.

10. Attribute everything you do in life to food and its associated evils. For example:
    - If you fail at work, remember that it is because your suit size is not the same as that of the waif sitting at reception, and because she is that size she will now get your job.
    - Oh yes, always remember that whenever someone stares at you it is because you are definitely the fattest thing they have ever seen in their lives.

11. If someone gives you a compliment, immediately assume that there is a hidden agenda: if you practise this often enough you will eventually realise that the compliment is meant to patronise you and make you feel bad.

12. If you don't lose according to the calorie-calculations, remember that you have now proven your body to be completely deformed,

and should not have been born in the first place. There could simply be no other reason for not losing any weight!

13. If you happen to eat something that brings you pleasure, immediately fill your brain with thoughts of guilt and come up with at least three plans on how to rid yourself of this evil: 3½ hours of spinning classes, then undress and examine exactly where it has gone to on your thighs, or ask your best friend for a copy of that three-day starvation diet (the pain of which you definitely deserve, by the way).

14. Each time you feel happy with your body, immediately replace the thought with: 'There is still someone out there thinner than me, therefore I am not a success.'

15. If, after trying everything, you still cannot lose weight, try the last option, for which there is much support offered: anorexia nervosa – it works.

I am being harshly ironic about 'the perfect diet' to show you the shocking reality of how we abuse our bodies. The consequences of mindless dieting are far-reaching and extremely dangerous. We often feel that we cannot control the incredibly strong attraction to food. This inability makes us vulnerable and often we relinquish control to ANYONE who is prepared to show us how to control our eating. So we become sheep under the staff of ruthless shepherds.

We condition ourselves to view food as the enemy – knowing that in fact we cannot live without it. Yet we spend huge amounts of money to slim, avoid social gatherings to hide our 'affliction' and nearly kill ourselves in the process. The tenacious succeed in doing just that, unfortunately.

7 FOOD OBSESSIONS: HOW COMMON ARE THEY?

Are you obsessed with food? Your first reaction to this question will probably be a vehement 'No!' Food obsession is a troublesome subject and it is understandable why we choose to avoid discussing it altogether. However, eating disorders are common, especially among women. Be brave, and read on.

There are two categories of people who are obsessive about food: those who immediately exempt themselves, and those who skilfully conceal their disorder.

The first group do not consider themselves obsessed with food at all. They listen patiently and politely when the criteria of food obsession are named, but disengage from further discussion. It is only when it becomes apparent that they meet many of the criteria themselves that they pay attention, recognising how distorted their perception of food has become.

The second group are those suffering from anorexia nervosa or bulimia nervosa. Their obsession with food is all-encompassing, but they artfully conceal their fixation. They may continue in this way for years, not admitting to the disorder. Only when they become too thin to escape notice, or take obvious measures to avoid food, will the disorder be revealed, unless the practised eye (and ear) of a well-trained therapist identify the tell-tale signs first. Anorexia, and how to treat it, will be discussed in detail in chapter 13.

DR DORA: How many eating disorders are there?

Most people have heard of bulimia and anorexia, but eating disorders do not end there. Many people have disordered eating patterns that do not fit the current strict diagnostic guidelines.

One area of intense research at present is 'Binge Eating Disorder',[1] This differs from bulimia because sufferers binge but do not purge. In other words, after a binge there is no vomiting, excessive exercise or use of laxatives. People with this condition have recurrent binges where several things happen:

- They eat large amounts of food in a short period of time
- They feel a lack of control while eating
- They often eat very quickly (without chewing)
- They end up feeling uncomfortably full
- They may not even start off by being hungry
- They often eat alone because they feel embarrassed
- The binge is followed by feelings of disgust, guilt and depression

To make a diagnosis, the bingeing must occur fairly regularly, at least two days a week for six months.

Most people suffering from this condition are women. They are frequently obese and have a lifetime history of depression.[2] An added problem it that they tend to have very disturbed sleep, even if they are not obese.[3]

This is not an obscure psychiatric diagnosis: bingeing is extremely common in women. An Austrian study indicated that over one in five women displayed some sort of bingeing behaviour.[4]

There are certain risks factors that predispose to developing binge eating disorder. Sadly, number one seems to be *dieting*.[5] One study examined 98 patients with binge eating disorder and found that for 65% of them, dieting had come first.[6]

Other risk factors identified by researchers are a history of traumatic childhood experiences as well as *parents* who were depressed. People who are repeatedly criticised about their shape, weight and eating habits may develop the disorder.

Some women who start off bingeing eventually end up vomiting, and bulimia develops. These women tend to be perfectionistic and have low self-esteem.[7]

The Austrian study mentioned above identified ongoing restrictive eating ('watching what you eat'), dieting and excessive exercise as additional risk factors for binge eating disorder[8]

Once a woman starts binge eating disorder, the likelihood is that she will develop obesity and depression later on in life. In another study of 30 obese women with the condition, most reported that they had begun bingeing during adolescence when they were of a *normal weight*. Obesity and depression tended to occur several years later.[9] It is therefore extremely important to treat bingeing as early as possible, to prevent these complications from developing. Unfortunately, this is easier said than done because of the secretive nature of the disorder.

Denial

The first group (those who deny their obsessions with food) is tricky to deal with. Members of this group are often more difficult to treat successfully because they genuinely believe that the way they think about food is normal. This is not surprising, since we have been subjected to negative indoctrination about food for years.

Borderline food obsessors in our practice often require psychological treatment before any dietary therapy can begin. I would like to repeat some of their comments. Do these sound familiar?

- 'Oh no, I'm not sure if I could eat all that pasta! That would seem gluttonous!'
- 'Oh no! I'm proud to say that I never drink soft drinks like Coke.'
- 'No, I don't eat the same food as my family; poor things, they aren't on diet'.
- 'I have tried every diet you've ever heard of!'
- 'Don't ask me what I ate yesterday, it was a bad day.'
- 'You should have seen what I ate yesterday, I completely lost control, I don't know what came over me!'
- When asked what your favourite food is, you reply, 'I love a big, fresh salad, and a chicken breast.'
- When you talk about the cheese burger you had yesterday, you shrink a little and give an embarrassed laugh.
- You find yourself talking to friends about how much you ate 'the other day'.
- You make excuses for eating crisps and chocolates, like 'I'm premenstrual' or 'I'm going to have this because I've had such an awful day,' or 'Just a small amount, please.'
- When offered delicious food, you gasp and say, 'I really shouldn't, but that looks so nice, I'll just have a teeny bit.'
- You describe the food you eat using words like 'a dash of...' or 'a scraping of...' or even try and avoid the subject altogether.
- You are embarrassed to eat in public, and say to yourself, 'I hope nobody notices that I am eating this; they'll wonder how someone like me could afford to eat such fattening food.'

And if you ...

- have most of the books ever published about dieting (hopefully this will be your last!)
- have been baffled by the many conflicting ideas about what is fattening and what is not, and are now not only confused but also afraid to eat

- only order salad when you eat out, one after the other
- feel a sense of guilt or failure after eating a lasagna
- think about food all the time, not just when you are hungry
- do other things to keep your mind off food
- have repetitive food choices
- have frequent cravings for 'forbidden foods'
- have control tricks with food, like always leaving something on the plate, or taking just less than you feel you want
- ever binge-eat
- ever eat in private or hide food
- know that you can't just have a small amount of anything – you will eat the whole slab of chocolate if you buy one, not just a few squares
- view any food as being 'naughty' or 'evil'.

Have you ever said or done any of the above?

DR DORA: Are you obsessed *and* addicted?

Many people with food addictions are also dependent on alcohol or drugs. There seems to be an 'addictive personality' at play here. One study found that both bulimics and anorexics have highly addictive personalities.[10] Many eating disordered people also exercise madly. Are they 'addicted' to exercise? A second study compared the psychological profiles of two groups of heavy exercisers: eating disordered people who were exercise-dependent (they used exercise to control or lose weight); and healthy people without an eating disorder (who exercised simply for the love of it). For those lucky people who were addicted to exercise *for its own sake*, there was no evidence of an addictive personality.

Those who were eating disordered *and* exercise-dependent were:

- addictive
- impulsive
- obsessed with body shape and weight
- frequently mentally ill
- suffering from poor self esteem.[11]

Well, you have some changing to do, because those thoughts indicate that you have an unhealthy and dysfunctional attitude towards food. You must change now! Changing is a slow process, not merely a matter of pushing these well-engrained thoughts to the back of your mind. Dysfunctional eating means denying that your natural hunger must be obeyed. But this can be very difficult to do, especially if you have dieted for many years.

Simply read on, and you'll feel a few shivers down your spine as you realise how ignorance about food has turned a hungry tummy into a permanently twisted one.

The hunger urge is extremely powerful. If we deny ourselves the satisfaction of food, then our need for food becomes an addiction. We all have a fair idea what drug addiction is. It is an insatiable need for a substance that produces powerfully pleasurable effects, so powerful that when the effect wears off, the user must have another fix. Regular fixes will satisfy the need, and the dose can remain constant, producing the same effect. But if the user goes without the drug for a longer period than usual, the need increases, requiring a larger fix than before. The same applies to food, but when we deny ourselves food we create an 'addictive' feeling towards it, because of our need for it. The less you eat, the greater will be the urge to eat.

You may question this analogy, but when we follow the path of calorie cutting, we see exactly how this happens. The only difference between addiction to drugs and addiction to food is that we can choose to make food addictive. If we restrict our intake by calorie-cutting, then our physical reactions mount to ensure that all of our being is geared to getting that food. This sounds like an addiction, but is simply a natural reaction of one's body, preventing us from starvation and death. If we eat regularly, and according to our body's natural hunger signals, then this stressful craving will not arise! If, however, we take it upon ourselves to actively ignore these signals, the body's starvation mechanism will ensure that every physical reaction is enabled, making it feel as though we are 'addicted' to the food. It's like breathing: if you try and hold your breath for too long, your entire body will start changing, making it desperate to get more oxygen, and do everything in its power to get that oxygen. Using this analogy, we can see that this reaction is not an addiction or even a craving, it is just the body telling us to jolly well make sure we get what we need, because what we have is not sufficient!

DR DORA: Food or opium?

Drug addicts and alcoholics generally have two major problems. Firstly, they need more and more of their substance to get the same effects. This is because drugs of abuse (including alcohol) change the receptors they bind to in the brain, making them less sensitive.

To create the same rush, you need to use more drug. Secondly, if an addict stops taking the drug, unbearable withdrawal symptoms result. So they get hooked. Drugs of abuse stimulate the brain's pleasure centre (mediated by dopamine, a neurotransmitter relative of serotonin) and the 'feel good' centre in the limbic system, which is mediated by serotonin.

Pushing up serotonin levels

Food does not cause addiction in the same way that drugs do; but there is a link between eating and addiction. Eating certain foods can increase brain serotonin. A powerful booster of brain serotonin is the drug ecstasy. While not as dramatic, eating certain carbohydrates without protein can do it too.[12] People who snack in this way may experience a brief improvement in mood, presumably due to increased serotonin levels.[13] Once the trick is discovered, they may search out carbohydrate-rich 'comfort' foods such as cake, chocolate and potato chips – all of these are rich in fat too – to boost mood. If they continue eating like this, they may ultimately binge to create the same serotonin boost.

Dopamine is also involved in the 'addictive nature' of food. A truly pleasurable eating experience is reinforced by dopamine, acting via the reward center. After a good meal, the satisfied feeling is mediated by dopamine, which has connections to the part of the brain that regulates feeding. Without dopamine (no 'satisfaction' after the 'action' of eating) there is little urge to eat. In one study, mice lacking dopamine became listless and ultimately died of starvation.[14]

A caveat: the carbohydrate craving hypothesis has been refuted by several papers written by psychologists.[15, 16]

The opiate connection

Did you know that the brain manufactures its own opiates? Endorphins and enkephalins belong to a family of opium-like neurotransmitters. These chemicals that the body produces itself, play a role in appetite, stress and addiction. There is some controversy about exactly what opiates do to appetite. To some extent, it depends on which opiate and which receptor is involved. Opiates decrease appetite if they are present in specific parts of the brain. Not surprisingly, anorexics have very low levels of these opiates when they are starving.[17] Once the anorexics have gained some weight, the levels increase. On the other hand, prolonged dieting and vomiting can also *increase* opiate levels. There is a theory that eating disordered people become 'addicted' to their behaviours and that they crave the high levels of opiates that are released when they diet or vomit.[18, 19] Even if these people feel embarrassed about their disordered eating patterns, the urge to have the 'endorphin high' makes them continue.

We are dependent on food. Without it we will die, as we would without water to drink and air to breathe. When there is adequate food available we eat just enough to feel satisfied. But when we are deprived of food (whether through famine or dieting – the body knows no difference), the drive to obtain sustenance becomes overwhelming. This is the body's natural protective response against starving to death, because we are resilient creatures of survival. This drive is hormonally based, as we will see later, but simply follow me here.

With food deprivation, the body becomes aggressive and desperate. All its functions urgently signal the need for food: hunger pangs, a rumbling tummy, inability to concentrate, feelings of unease, headaches, even light-headedness and mild tremors. This unpleasant and all-encompassing sensation drives us to find food. But again, it is the fact that we have restricted to the point of hunger and mild depression that causes our bodies to need to eat and return to normal again! So: don't calorie-restrict if you want your body to be totally in control of itself!

DR DORA: Hungry anorexics

There is an interesting mistake in psychiatry: the use of the word anorexia in describing the illness anorexia nervosa. In medical jargon, anorexia means 'loss of appetite'. This does not happen to anorexics! They remain hungry, however much they restrict their diets.

In addition to cutting down on food intake, anorexics display a variety of peculiar behaviours around food. However, it is true that anorexics feel 'full' after eating very little. This has also been described in starving people.

Let's take it one step further. When dieting you will be aware of these unpleasant sensations, but might employ one or more of the many coping mechanisms in order not to respond to them. For instance, taking appetite suppressants or bulking agents; drinking vast amounts of fluids; changing your routine; avoiding social situations where there may be food; doing more exercise, etc. These techniques may be effective for a short while, but the body's mechanisms are too sensitive to be fooled by our 'tricks'. The urge to eat will return, and this time stronger than before. You have now become obsessed with food, but the dieting specialist has told you that this is part of the process, and that you must persist.

A day in the life of a dieter

I wonder if the following sounds familiar to you?

You have embarked on a diet because you feel too fat. A friend recommended that you consult with her 'diet guru' who has had great success in helping people lose weight quickly. He suggested a spartan eating plan, and although it seems very little to eat, you are motivated to lose the weight.

At work one morning you feel quite hungry. You experience the normal signs of hunger: your tummy rumbles and you feel distinct hunger pangs, you find it difficult to concentrate and your head aches dully. Soon you begin to feel slightly uneasy and become light-headed.

The guru said these symptoms are normal and easily controllable. He was adamant that you should not satisfy these urges, no matter how strong they are. As the intensity of the hunger pangs renders you weak and ready to succumb to the urge to eat, so your self-esteem starts to plummet. Your headache gets worse and you start to tremble.

(I hope that while you are reading this, you are acutely aware of how much this need for food is rapidly turning into an obsession/ addiction.)

Taking an appetite suppressant and a few headache pills, you try to continue with your work. After a while, the sandwich trolley passes and your feelings of anxiety increase. You consider ways to 'cheat' the system, rationalising how 'just a little bit' won't make much of a difference.

DR DORA: The dangers of appetite suppressants

Taking tablets to cut appetite may start an addiction, cause severe anxiety or even life-threatening high blood pressure. Yet many of these drugs are available without a prescription. Most appetite suppressants are stimulants, in the same class as amphetamine (speed). They are bad news!

You have a choice: eat, or ignore the urge for food. But because the guru said not to give in, you take the latter course. As you attempt to work, your body's urgent demand for food gets stronger.

The food on the trolley haunts you – images fill your mind and regardless of how hard you try, you can't stop obsessing. By this stage you will feel quite strange and almost out of control. Food was never this important before, but now you are obsessing about the stuff! What on earth has happened?

You recall the fellow dieters at the guru's office. They lost weight successfully – they were strong enough to ignore these thoughts and needs. You have to be strong too.

But these feelings are powerful! When your colleagues unwrap their sandwiches the smell is overwhelming. Grumpy and ratty now, you feel deprived. You are also angry because you have allowed yourself to gain this much weight. Everyone but you seems to have a normal appetite; everyone but you is in control. You feel like a fat pig, and think that you deserve to go through this agony …

As the days go by you become increasingly unpleasant and irritable. You feel completely devoid of willpower and seem to yourself totally out of control. Because you can't stop thinking about food, you employ other self-hating techniques to frighten yourself away from food, and in the direction of the guru's perception of how thin you should be. You stick a photograph of your 'fat self' on the fridge door. Now any thought of 'cheating' will be foiled when you see that repulsive fat woman. You think about having a small piece of chocolate. But why the sudden craving for chocolate? Before, you would have a piece after dinner and think no more of it, now you want to drive to the store to buy a whole slab! What is happening?

You feel stupid to have walked around like this for so long! The guru said you have to lose 10kg. How embarrassing! You briefly consider surgery. With your head throbbing, you reach for the diet sheet to check on your daily allowance. Two savoury biscuits in an hour's time … that hardly seems enough! You start wondering whether it's all worth the effort. No one else appears to go through this much agony!

You rationalise that the guru knows what he's talking about and that you deserve to suffer like this because you are fat. How ugly you look in the photo stuck on the fridge. The tremors become worse as your hunger increases, but the guru said to distract yourself …

If only you could stop thinking about food. You feel useless and weak when you compare yourself to the other strong-willed dieters. If you forfeit the biscuits being passed around the tea-room, you will feel strong again – even stronger if you forfeit a whole meal. Then the guru will be pleased. You won't be embarrassed to step on the scale next time.

Your thoughts turn to your matric dance. How slim you were! Things seemed so much better then. You never felt this unhappy and you always had a normal appetite. Again it seems as if your body and mind have reeled out of control.

It's time for a weigh-in. The guru will be waiting. Fervently hoping that you've lost, you approach the hated scale. You really want to prove that you are a good dieter, that you can be strong if you want to. You didn't cheat this week, but you are premenstrual and that means being bloated with water …

Stayed the same! Stayed the same! Oh no!

Firstly you consider the guru's reaction. He probably thinks that you've been cheating! You know that you haven't, but the look in his eye says he does not believe you. You feel that your body has failed you again. You HATE your body …

The guru adapts your diet plan. He suggests that you eat less than before, but to show him that you can lose weight, you will eat even less than that, until your stupid body works properly. You find it hard to believe that losing weight is so difficult this time. Previously you lost significantly, but then you were a bit younger. You resign yourself to the fact that as your body gets older you will never be able to eat normally again.

You hate feeling out of control. To relax, you watch TV. Wrong choice! The advertisements are all about food, one after the other … So many of them, all featuring people eating. Seething, you think that it is only a matter of time before they will get fat like you. If they can eat like that, they deserve to suffer like you … But maybe they won't, you think. Again the feelings of insecurity strike. Maybe it is because you are useless and your body is awkwardly shaped …

You consider joining the gym. You cannot really afford the contract, but the promise of achieving a figure like the skinny young girls in sexy gym gear motivates you to join anyway. If you looked like them, everybody might accept you, especially your husband. Come to think of it, things haven't been so good between the two of you lately. You've been giving him the cold shoulder for a while now, thinking that he doesn't want to see you like this. You also resent him, because you know he doesn't think about food all day!

Even though you are tired to the bone because you are eating so little, you join an aerobics class at the gym, thinking that the exercise might be torture enough to teach you a lesson about food. Even if you can't keep up with the instructor, it will be your penance for being useless.

Fatigue racks your body. The mere thought of even trying to start the exercises scares you. Hating yourself more and more, you consider giving it all up. What's the point of being good? Besides, you're sick to death of thinking about food all the time …

I hope you are as exhausted as I am by reading this! But it's too common to hide. Perhaps much of it has touched you before! Just pause for a moment: can you think of ONE reason why this doesn't sound like an addiction?

Trying to live on a strict calorie reduced diet plays havoc with a person's self-worth and pride. This usually continues as the dieter remains consumed with self-loathing. The end result is a complicated, unhappy, aggressive, defensive and desperate woman.

Stop it! Just stop it! Dieting is NOT something that just anyone can do. It is DIFFICULT. It is NOT a matter of merely eating less. We have to change our perceptions about food!

New perceptions

Firstly, we have to relax about food. Most people find this really hard to do. I use the story of our dog, a stray, to help them understand. When we fed her for the first time after getting her from the SPCA, she bolted the food down. We were amazed that it actually stayed down.

This continued night after night, until gradually she realised that she was never going to starve again. She knew that there would always be the same amount of food presented to her as she wanted it, day after day, and so her eating became more relaxed, and less urgent or obsessive.

As a dog on the streets, her entire psyche was geared to panic-eat if and when there was food, which was not often. If initially we had increased the size of her meals, she would not have known when to stop because her brain had long forgotten the satiety signals indicative of plenty. Now that she has no fear of starvation, she glances nonchalantly at her food, sniffs around in a relaxed manner, and then eats until she has had enough, at which point she happily trots off without a second thought.

This story illustrates how instinctive this all-or-nothing food relationship is when we starve ourselves. It cannot be controlled consciously or in any other way. The power of the hunger drive is completely beyond the human mind. The more we attempt to control it by removing ourselves from the temptation of food, the more our bodies physiologically retaliate by increasing the drive. It is, after all, our number one physiological and instinctual survival technique, and it works very well.

DR DORA: What is satiety?

Satiety is a sensation that tells us that we are satisfied, full and can stop eating. Control of appetite is very complex and involves several brain areas.[20] The hypothalamus is constantly monitoring the nutritional state of the body. It keeps tabs on blood glucose and fat levels and gets instructions from circulating hormones and neurotransmitters.[21] After a meal is over, the digestive system and fat cells signal to the hypothalamus that they are 'satisfied' and the conscious part of the brain 'tells' us to stop eating.

Of the neurotransmitters playing a part in the control of appetite, serotonin is critical. High serotonin levels are linked to satiety,[22] whereas low serotonin levels increase appetite. Women with bulimia nervosa tend to have low serotonin levels whereas in anorexics they are actually high.[23] One of the many theories of why people develop eating disorders is that the satiety centre in the hypothalamus is not functioning correctly. Either there is too little serotonin acting on the hypothalamus, so the person is never satiated and binges (as in bulimia). Or the serotonin levels are abnormally high and the feeling of satiety persists, even in the face of starvation (anorexia).

As we have discussed before, there is an intimate link between serotonin level and carbohydrate craving. High serotonin levels tell the hypothalamus to stop us eating starchy foods (but have little effect on how much fat or protein we eat).[24] This is because the more carbohydrate we eat, the more serotonin is synthesised. The hypothalamus 'switches off' serotonin production after a carbohydrate-rich meal by telling us to stop eating!

Regardless of our space-age technology and medical hypotheses, humans cannot transcend this primeval instinct. We have tried to master our instincts, but the consequences were disastrous to body and mind equally.

We should stop taking the black-and-white option in thinking that we can control this monumentally complex body of ours with a simple plus/minus equation of calories. How conceited of us! Calorie-cutting is not the solution to the battle of the bulge.

It is difficult to just **stop** obsessing about food when we are still following a restrictive diet – we have to adopt a whole new style of eating to prevent ever again becoming obsessed about food.

We have to stop calorie restricting NOW and move ahead to become healthy, lean, happy and stable!

Remember, your body is unaware that it lives in the 21st century and that it is being wilfully starved in order to look like a gaunt supermodel. The human body has been fine-tuned over thousands of years to survive through periods of feast and famine. It can carefully monitor the number of 'famines' it has endured, and will make sure that when food becomes available again, it 'stockpiles', ready for the next famine. The human body has developed the most powerful physical and mental or emotional resources over time to protect it against death by starvation. These are deeply ingrained in the psyche, and will obviously make it incredibly difficult, if not impossible, to eat the minute quantities of food prescribed by 'traditional' starvation techniques to lose weight and to maintain weight.

Restrictive diets do not work!

HOW CALORIE RESTRICTING LEADS TO CLINICAL DEPRESSION

8

Share with me the joys of a fresh loaf of bread, still warm from the bakery ...

As you take it from the packet, the heady aroma of steamy, risen yeast is released. You slice through the crust and the softness of the loaf yields to your touch and sinks below the knife. With fingers moist from the steam, you spread honey over its supple surface. Glossy sweetness sinks slowly and seductively and where cold meets hot, a contrast of golden clarity mingles to form the perfect fusion of fla-vours. As the first bite enters your eager mouth, it ignites a blissful sensation. The sticky nectar slips around your tongue and the rush of expectation is satisfied. You close your eyes as the flavours and textures mingle. It feels as if fulfilment is dissolving into your blood. Your heart beats warmer and your body relaxes as you reach the plateau of ultimate contentment.

All this from a slice of bread and honey? Yes! This is why taste buds were made so sensitive. Moreover, the taste buds are also inex-tricably linked with the emotional side of the brain. In fact, the signals coming from your taste buds stimulate so many responses in the body that it is sacrilege to deny yourself their pleasurable effects!

In truth, the good feelings you get from carbohydrates actually have a physiological basis. Remember when you eat carbohydrates that dissolve quickly into your system? They fill up the blood with sugar until insulin pushes it out and stores it in the muscles. For that brief moment, while sugar levels are high, the serotonin pro-duced increases substantially.

Remember serotonin – the feel-good, tempering and calming chemical in your brain? Well, the production of serotonin is stimulated when blood sugar levels increase. This is why you crave carbohydrates (especially the fast-releasing ones like bread, potatoes, cane sugar, corn flakes and rice crispies). A craving is your body's signal that either your sugar levels are too low and must be rectified immediately, or that the serotonin function is amiss (there isn't enough or you are not feeling its effects enough). That is also why a lot of these fast-dissolving sugars have been affectionately known as 'comfort foods'. That is exactly what they do for you: they comfort you physically and emotionally.

Long-gone are the words 'empty calories' to describe refined sugars. People used to think they were wasteful calories that did not provide nutrients to nourish the body. This is like saying that you shouldn't wear perfume because it contains no active healing properties! I mean, perfume is a luxury we enjoy because of our need to feel lovely. We do not need perfume to survive; there's nothing about it to suggest that it is even good for you. But, most of us make sure a few sprays go on each morning – because it's nice. That's all. And life is supposed to be filled with nice little things. The same holds for sugar.

But, if all you ever have is sugar, sugar, sugar, your taste buds may be very happy, but exclusion of all the other important foods in the diet will lead to deficiency-related disorders that are very damaging. A diet of only sugar and sticky buns will lead to disease. Although it provides lots of energy it is not balanced with nutritious foods. This sticky bun diet will not provide vitamins, minerals or fibre, and so constipation, cancer and diseases of imbalance will ensue. Imbalance is the problem, not sugar.

However, adding sugar and bread to an already nutritious and varied diet simply puts the attractive cherry on top. It makes nutritious and delicious foods even better than they already are. So add these little sparkles to the diet, do not replace it with them.

Getting back to the effect food has on neurotransmitters (brain chemicals). You have seen how high levels of sugar in the blood stimulate production of serotonin, the feel-good signal. This is integral to well-being and now you can understand why the body 'self-medicates' with high GI (fast-releasing) carbohydrates when it runs short of serotonin.

The complication is that it is often not clear what came first, the chicken or the egg. Does the serotonin level go down for some reason, and so you crave sugars? Or does it work the other way round: you cut out carbohydrates, and so your serotonin levels drop? From my experience, both occur simultaneously, as a result of calorie cutting.

DR DORA: Dieting, serotonin and depression

We have discussed how prolonged dieting might lead to an eating disorder. How commonly does depression arise from restrictive dieting? Can you starve yourself into depression? These are very complex questions and we certainly do not have all the answers. It does appear that serotonin is implicated in both depression and unsuccessful dieting.[1]

Let us go back to the very beginning of serotonin production: tryptophan. We have seen how the neurotransmitter serotonin is synthesised from a protein building block called tryptophan. When we eat certain proteins, we obtain tryptophan from the diet. Small amounts of it can also be manufactured inside the liver. To complicate the picture further, it appears that eating certain combinations of proteins – without trytophan – can decrease serotonin production.[2] On the other hand, eating high carbohydrate meals *without protein* may increase serotonin production.[3]

Many studies have examined the role of tryptophan in mood disorders. There are two questions:

- If tryptophan is eliminated from the diet, is less serotonin produced and are people therefore prone to depression?
- If depressed people are given tryptophan to eat, does it lift mood?
- Depleting the diet of tryptophan lowers mood and causes brain waves to slow down.[4] In experiments, it is easy to deplete the body of tryptophan by replacing the normal, balanced diet by one that includes an amino acid mixture *without tryptophan.* Immediately, tryptophan levels in the blood and brain drop.[5] As a result, the production and release of serotonin decrease.[6] Even if depressives have been treated with medication and are feeling happy again, suddenly removing tryptophan from their diets causes them to sink back into a temporary depressed state.[7, 8, 9] As yet, there are no reports in the scientific literature of *prolonged* depression following tryptophan depletion.
- Increasing dietary tryptophan has been shown to improve mild depression.

Eating a *high carbohydrate-low protein* diet improves depression. An interesting study gave one group of subjects a carbohydrate-rich meal and the other group a protein-rich meal. Both groups were exposed to a stressful situation. The people who had eaten the carbohydrates were protected against depression and high cortisol levels (the stress hormone). They also performed well intellectually. Those who ate the high protein meal showed a deterioration in mood, cortisol level and intellect.[10]

Depressed people seem to want to protect themselves against low serotonin levels by eating lots of carbohydrate. Another study examined the diets of depressed versus non-depressed people.[11] As you might have guessed, the depressives ate more carbohydrates whereas the normal controls ate more protein. Other aspects of their diets were similar. It is not surprising that when we feel down, we crave carbohydrates.

If you have read ***The X-Diet***, then you will be familiar with my own rapid descent into an eating disorder. And in my practice I have treated many serious eating disorders and depressives, and have seen how dieting was a big trigger for them as well. Let me talk you through a typical dieting scenario, and you will recognise how the serotonin drops rapidly and uncontrollably.

You may wake up one morning and think, 'Time to diet'. After all, it is clear as the light of day reflecting off the glossy cover of a dieting magazine that the only way to prevent obesity is to eat less – much less – than normal. So you start dieting. Bleating obediently, faithfully following the information in the magazine, you reduce the 'fattening' carbohydrates. It doesn't take a brain surgeon to deduce what happens to your blood sugar levels. They drop. They drop steadily, and slowly, and your body almost gets used to this low sugar level; never really filling up at all. When the blood sugar levels remain 'below par', what happens to the serotonin production? It will also drop! So, you feel the first hints of depressed serotonin function already: lethargy, short-temper, irritability, anxiety and … cravings!

Of course! Do you think your body likes being like this? If you deprive your body of sleep for several nights, won't it automatically make the need for sleep almost uncontrollable? And if you are silly enough to further ignore these fine-tuned signals, won't you turn into a short-fused, slightly hysterical banshee? Of course you will! Your body is much stronger than your silly willpower! Don't mess with nature! It knows best.

So, the cravings, irritability, anxiety and unease increase to a slightly surreal pitch. Now your body realises it is in for a battle for survival. All the other physiological tricks switch on during this time. Remember what happens when you eat fewer calories than you are burning up? Your body starts a process of auto-cannibalisation, and the by-products of this are ketones, which circulate in the blood and start the ketotic psychosis. This is a state of false euphoria, possibly a successful method of self-preservation during periods of famine. It comprises feelings of euphoria, energy, lack of hunger, and overall well-being. Much like cocaine, from what I hear. Sounds good, but it signifies that the body is losing weight too quickly, and muscle is being auto-cannibalised to a lower metabolism (see chapter 10 for details).

DR DORA: What are ketones?

Ketones are made in the liver and are used by the body as an energy source when glucose is not readily available. Ketones are always present in the blood and their levels increase during fasting and prolonged exercise. They are also found in the blood of neonates and pregnant women.[12]

High levels of ketones may have some effect on mental state, but exactly what that is has not been well-described. 'Ketotic psychosis' is not a psychiatric term.

Your serotonin levels are dropping; thus removing your calm, rational thought processes. And you exacerbate the whole thing by increasing the ketones in your blood! This turns you into an obsessive, irrational, desperate and excess-driven witch – so typical of a dieter. Rabidly searching for ways to further 'trick' your body, you buy pills that drug you further from appetite than you already are.

And your life begins to suffer. The lack of serotonin means that your cravings for sugars are now stronger than ever, and you are pushed further and further into the abyss of discord and emotional anarchy.

If this lasts long enough, you will have feelings of failure and lack of control and may enter a struggle to assert conscious control over what you see as your hedonistic bodily instincts. The feeling of being slave to your impulses and primitive instincts can break down your sense of personal integrity.

After much calorie restriction, and over a long time, clinical depression is bound to follow. We've now seen how. I am not referring here to an emotional depression, which needs comfort, love and support. I am talking about a more serious chemical imbalance: dysfunctional brain control and imbalanced chemicals. These are clinical, psychiatric disorders, whose symptoms are deemed acceptable if performed under the pious auspices of 'weight control'.

ENOUGH! Enough, I say!

Let's stop. Think. Understand. And heal. It's about time we start to appreciate our bodies for what they are and realise that these feelings and desires are simply an abused body returning to its deepest and most primeval survival techniques, and protecting us from death! Our bodies are temples, and are meant to be preserved; to be worshipped; to be marvelled at. Not to be fought and belittled by an obsession for complete tyrannical control by the mind. After all, we cannot possibly separate the body and the mind, no matter how hard we try. The brain is still a functioning organ, controlled by the status of the body, and vice versa.

Attempts to control natural urges (as if signals from the brain don't exist), lead to the anorexic phobia of not wanting to be in the body; not wanting to be at the mercy of natural bodily functions;

hating what cannot be controlled by the mind as it confirms the notion of the 'developed mind trapped inside the physical, urge-driven being'.

So enters the pattern:

- Starve, and serotonin levels drop.
- Feel out of control with these new, strong cravings, and sacrifice further.
- Hate the natural bodily instincts that prevent you from achieving success and from controlling your mind. But ... the more you remove yourself from the body's screams, the louder it screams.

Food is now seen as a life or death choice:

- If you choose to eat, your mind will have failed you by succumbing to the person you are competing against the most – your physical being. You will have given in to your body's base and uncontrollable desires that constantly plague you.
- By choosing not to eat, you will have conquered this physical need. You will have won, because this monstrous creature of need, desire and lust (your body) will diminish by the day.

Because you have not allowed yourself to give in to your instincts, you view yourself as successful and supremely above nature. The mind is as powerful as you want it to be ... You ARE in control. You ARE in control. YOU ARE IN CONTROL.

Listen to the voice in your mind: 'My uncontrolled physical urges are so strong that they are my greatest fear. If you gave me chocolate, I would eat 12! So, don't give me a chocolate at all! If it's not there, it can't harm me ...'

You think that stopping this control would render you a failure, joining the 'fatso's' who are completely at the mercy of their base desires. People who have no control. NO, you think! You will not be like that! You will not be seen as a gluttonous pig! You will not allow yourself to eat! You will not show how your body controls you. You are in control.

The body only ever spins out of control when it is forced to, like when it is starved. Then it is forced it back into instinctual patterns of survival. It also relinquishes control when you show no signs of 'moderation'. Moderation is taboo for someone in this state, because living in moderation means that the body is *not* out of control. But this body *is* out of control. Moderation, for this person, is impossible. It is all or nothing; succeed or fail. There can be no in-betweens; it is too risky.

This happens when the neurotransmitter (serotonin) – which gives one control to live in the 'grey' area and not swing to the destructive black-or-white extremes – is the very substance that has been depleted by restricting carbohydrate intake. To stop the cycle is the difficult part. To get such a person to eat carbohydrates at this stage is almost impossible. Now carbohydrates cannot increase serotonin, because the very lack of serotonin has rendered the brain irrational, refusing all food.

You have to realise that calorie cutting nudges you into a spiral of self-destruction from which you may not be able to escape (depending on your life circumstances and initial mental health). And once you are in this serotonin 'depression', it becomes vital to have parameters; but parameters laid down by someone else. Someone to tell you how much of this; not that much of that; this weight of that, etc.

In this state of depression you need these parameters, for without them, this new uncontrollable body will not know when to stop. It now controls you.

DR DORA: Do you choose how you look from what you eat?

We look the way we do because of genetic factors as well as what we eat. Clearly, the kind of diet we prefer influences our body shape. Our genes interact with the environment to produce the final outcome – our reflection in the mirror.

So what are the behavioural patterns that influence body shape? These involve the kinds of foods we select to eat as well as how much we eat and exercise. Researchers have divided human eating patterns into two distinct groups: low fat and high fat. The amount of fat a person consumes is the strongest predictor for weight gain, but it does not predict that an individual will be obese. In other words, it is not a simple equation that decides the more fat we eat equals the more fat laid down in our bodies. In a study of young men who ate either low or high fat diets, there were differences in appetite, basal metabolic rate, heart rate and how quickly the body digested fat and starch.[13] So weight control depends to a certain degree on what we choose to eat, but there is more complexity involved.

But these parameters laid down by the 'guru' we described earlier require you to take your miniature scale along to weigh portions when you eat out and to know the calorie content of everything you eat. In this state of depression you have to be told how much you may eat.

You will feel that this body that exercised such control once, is now nothing more than a puppet to your uncontrollable lusts. So now you are unable to set your own parameters of moderation: You have proven that you are incapable of doing this. The guru was right, you do need him and his parameters. Whatever he says you will do. He knows best, you know nothing. Every week you must go to be measured and to receive your dose of control. You are completely out of control, and you will join the other disciples, obediently bouncing between the boundaries he sets. Only then will you be safe from obesity ...

What are we doing to ourselves, and where do we go from here?

Once you have reached this point of almost no return, you will have to consult a physician, a psychiatrist and a dietician to help you get well again. However, the objective of this book is to educate, so that you never have to descend into this hell.

- Firstly, acknowledge that dieting can, and does kill!
- Secondly, understand the physiological workings of your body, and stop fighting it.

The quickest way to weaken a person into submission is by starvation and confinement to a mindless routine. Some know this as a concentration camp, but to women this is willpower!

9

HOW DIETING CAN LEAD TO AN EATING DISORDER

Having less food means having less of everything – literally. You have less fun, less energy, less taste, less satisfaction, less health and less happiness. When you eat too little, the brain chemicals alter to achieve a more energy-conserving state, i.e. depression.

Whilst depression often ensues during strict dieting, the metabolism slows down as well, for reasons of auto-adaptation and survival. So, without realising it, you become a victim of an out-of-control metabolism as well as of depressed mood.

This is the common fate of dieters, and one of the many reasons why dieting doesn't work. The body's natural and powerful instincts and reactions cannot be altered on a long-term basis. Its physical adaptation processes are so well rehearsed and powerful that they occur involuntarily, regardless. The more you attempt to control them, the more the body fights back to retain those functions in order to survive.

Consider it for a while. The body is an unbelievable feat of nature. It is a living, functioning product shaped by nature over thousands of years. How can we mere mortals think that weighing every scrap of food before eating it will beat the system for good? It seems a bit presumptuous, doesn't it?

Let's look at the way calorie-cutting effects physical and psychological changes to the brain. Have another fat-free muffin with extra jam, because this journey requires a lot of serotonin and energy!

This is the story of Ann, an ordinary, lovely young woman. At 17, she is of a normal size and appearance. Surprisingly normal, in fact. She wears a size 34 clothing, and wants to study law after school. She plays squash twice a week, likes trendy clothes and enjoys going to the movies. Paul, her boyfriend, thinks she is very pretty, with a great sense of humour to boot. Her life is uncomplicated and happily normal.

Lately, conversations at school revolve mainly around dieting, and what not to eat. Her friends say things like, 'Look at my thighs' or 'Ugh, my bum is getting so huge', even though their thighs and bums look quite normal. They all seem to have different ideas about what makes them fat and how best to get thin – information mostly obtained from women's magazines.

Ann listens quietly, not knowing how to participate in the conversation. She has always considered her figure adequate, but perhaps she's missing something. At home she thinks about the issue. She is certain that Paul has no problem with her figure; he has never said anything to the contrary.

During the next few days at school, her awareness about size suddenly becomes more acute. As she and her friends page through women's magazines she looks at the models. In fact, she's never really noticed before, but those girls whom everyone considers to be really beautiful, are also extremely thin. Moreover, as they discuss the models, there seems to be more giggles about Hannah, the 'fat' girl of the class. Hannah doesn't seem popular at all.

The penny drops. Her friends must be conveying an indirect message: she is too fat! Fat equals unsuccessful – she has to lose weight. She cringes with embarrassment. How could she have been happy with her figure, she worries; it's obvious to them that it is far from perfect.

Ann is a dedicated student and knows that hard work guarantees success. Average is not good enough. Her master plan for the future is set. She has no reason not to perform well. She is bright, young and full of energy, and knows that she can achieve whatever she puts her mind to. Shedding the extra weight must now slot into her plan and she will succeed with that too. Simple.

Apprehensively she searches magazines for a way to get thin. Just average body-size does not show success! She finds a diet, deciding that it looks simple enough. "Lose 4 kg in 1 week!" the caption promises. Stepping onto the bathroom scale, she holds her breath as the needle wavers back and forth, and settles on....58kg. She wonders what her friends weigh, and can't wait to find out.

The next day at school is filled with the novelty of dieting. It is an adult concept that gives her an exciting feeling of control. This is her plan; something she can do by herself and succeed at without help. Now she can contribute to the fashionable self-admonishment that her friends practise. 'Look at my waist!' she exclaims in disgust as she reaches for the packed tuna salad lunch, 'Thank heavens the diet will get rid of it soon.'

While talking Ann notices for the first time that her tummy is actually rounded. According to her friends a tummy should recede below the hipbones when lying on one's back. Hers doesn't do that. Fortunately she is doing something about it! How embarrassing not to have noticed this before. While she was under the impression that her figure was acceptable, everyone else could clearly see that it wasn't. Sure, her tummy isn't gross, but it certainly isn't anything to be proud of! How naïve she had been.

The next few days on the diet are fine. Her tummy certainly starts feeling quite hollow. She lies on her back each day to check whether it has receded below her hipbones yet and notices with pleasure that it seems to be getting there.

She really does feel quite hungry, though. It would be nice to finish the diet and to have a normal meal again. But, she remembers, she has to stay in control. All her friends do. And besides, childhood eating is over – controlling one's appetite is what women do.

When Ann weighs herself a week later she is overjoyed: 56kg! She has done it; proven to herself that she can control her appetite and change the shape of her body!

But according to the magazine she should have lost 4kg, so she must keep going for one week longer. 'This is easy,' she thinks as she skips off the scale – this newly discovered power makes her feel very special indeed, as does the knowledge that control and discipline gets results!

The following week Ann's lunch box is filled with more dry tuna salad and while the rest of the family enjoys a nice dinner; her meal consists of boiled fish. They are old-fashioned and small-minded, she thinks. They live in cocoons, not caring about their looks.

It would have been considerate if someone had told her earlier that she was fat, she muses. She really does miss the nice food, but she does not deserve it yet. Just 2kg to go ...

She weighs herself daily now, but there is hardly any change. Her body seems to be failing her, although she has followed the diet to the last letter. As the two-week mark looms closer, she worries that she will not lose the remaining kilograms. She decides to eat even less for the next few days to teach her 'greedy' body a lesson.

Two days later the 2kg have been shed. However Ann feels strangely aggressive towards her body – it had failed her and she had to teach it a lesson by almost starving. She knows that it was on the verge of getting out of control. In case this ever happened again, she has to remove the temptation of food properly.

Although she weighs 54kg (her goal), she wonders whether she is still too heavy for her height. After some inquiries she learns that for her height she should weigh between 53 and 58kg. Middle-of-the-road isn't good enough – she needs to weigh 52kg to have some leeway, to be better than just acceptable. She was actually overweight before! Well, certainly overweight for someone who is going to be a part of the 'better' part of society! Part of being acceptable means not letting your body go to pot!

She continues to eat even less. The hunger pangs get worse. She battles to sleep and lies awake at night, dreaming about food. During the day pervasive thoughts of food disturb her concentration. She argues with her mother who demands that she eat her rice and potatoes because she needs the energy! Ann explains that there is plenty of energy on her thighs and rudely accuses her mum of being negligent in allowing her to get so fat in the first place.

It is obvious to her that her mother simply does not understand that times have changed – that women can't be rounded and 'motherly' any more. They have to be thin to show their power and control.

Hunger pursues her relentlessly. Ann has to find ways of preventing herself from succumbing to her 'animal urge' to pig out. The mirror becomes her enemy. Disgustedly, she observes her 'fat' parts (those that were acceptable to her before). This is what everyone else sees, she thinks. She is fat and needs to lose more weight! She compares herself to the pictures in the magazines repeatedly. Those girls definitely don't weigh 52 kg – they look more like 48kg or less!

To ensure that she is acceptable to society, she decides to slim down to 47kg. The magazines are important. Never again can she trust her own judgement of her physique when she had been so horribly wrong! Her body distorts things, she broods. It tells her that everything is fine, but this just isn't true.

One evening as she sits down she notices that her tummy is still not concave. Her goal seems so far off, she feels desperate and starts to cry. Then the tears turn to anger at her weakness. Her friends certainly wouldn't cry for food, they are strong! But her pig-like craving for food is detestable. Her body isn't normal – it needs to be controlled. She knows that each time she relaxes her vigil she wants to eat, and if she eats, she will grow into a gross, fat slob. It is obvious to her that her body won't allow her to lose weight because it is totally out of control. No matter what she eats, Ann thinks, she will gain weight. After all, if it won't budge now when she's eating so little, can you imagine what will happen if she ever eats a normal meal again? Had her friends not shown her how easily the female body loses control, she would have grown like an elephant!

Ann is constantly hungry and cold. And angry. All her friends diet with such apparent ease; they never seem to be hungry. Disgusted, she regards her own failure. Why was she given this stupid body that is so obsessed with food and eating?

She turns her anger toward Paul. Even he is dumb and old-fashioned to have thought that her figure was agreeable. Now he says that she is getting too thin. Too thin for what, she wonders morosely. Probably for a housewife ... But Ann has greater aspirations than that and the man she eventually marries will only want the best. And being the best means being in control; showing her body how to be normal.

She spends long periods resentfully inspecting herself in the mirror to remind her of how fat she is. She has become extremely emotional, crying without reason and displaying irrational aggression in general. Constantly her thoughts turn to food, her concentration wanes and she becomes forgetful of most things.

Ann realises that her urge to eat is more powerful than she had ever expected. To avoid succumbing to her 'animal urges' she reminds herself constantly how ugly she is, how abhorrent her urges are and how undeserving of anything pleasurable she is.

In her efforts to avoid 'failing', she barters with herself, 'allowing' herself pleasures only if she loses more weight, or eats less. Denying herself all pleasures is the way she punishes herself for never quite reaching 47kg. She even invents reasons for her perceived unworthiness and displeasure, and then fools herself into believing them to be true.

By punishing herself in this way her self-hatred is fuelled, and when she hates herself, it prevents her from eating. She interprets compliments as a disguised and weak attempts at making her feel better; lies told by those who want to control her, jealous of her 'success' in losing weight. Resolutely she refuses to give in. Their 'well-meaning sweetness' is quite transparent to her, and infuriating. Their actions mirror those of her body: trying all sorts of tricks to get her to fail.

Heedless of the imminent danger to her body and soul, Ann will stay in control. She may have, however, reached a point of no return ...

It is evident from the above that Ann has spiralled into the beginnings of an eating disorder – anorexia nervosa. At this point either anorexia continues, meaning that she will continue eating less and less, or she will become bulimic, which implies binge eating and purging.

The bulimic hates herself into submission, and repeatedly tests her own willpower. She will continue with the destructive pattern of self-hatred, which fuels the strength to stay away from food. The psychiatric symptoms here relate to the serotonergic system: she displays obsessiveness, severe and ongoing anxiety, self-loathing, disturbed sleep patterns, irritability, poor concentration and memory. She desperately fears being out of control.

One of the main reasons for her obsessive thoughts of food is her body's overwhelming physiological need to eat! By restricting her intake, her serotonin production may initially have decreased. However, once the eating disorder is established, serotonin levels are high, which decreases appetite.

DR DORA: The challenge of anorexia nervosa

Anorexia nervosa remains a baffling disorder with the highest mortality rate of all psychiatric illnesses.[1] It occurs predominantly in adolescents and is 10-20 times commoner in girls than in boys.

While we are beginning to understand how appetite is regulated, very few inroads have been made with respect to the *causes* of anorexia. Most psychiatric disorders involve a combination of biological, psychological and social factors; and this is especially true of anorexia. In understanding these factors, much work remains to be done. Even the name of the disease is a misnomer. As we mentioned in Chapter 2, the word anorexia means 'loss of appetite'. But anorexics remain hungry and continue to diet despite persistent starvation.

From a sociological point of view, in every generation a standard is set for female beauty. There does seem to be a link between what the prevailing culture determines as the 'desirable woman' and what kind of eating disorders predominate. Our current society's obsession with *thinness* may be a factor in the prevalence of anorexia in teenage girls.[2]

Apart from this societal influence, genetic factors may also play a role in the development of the illness. Identical twins, who share the same genetic material, show higher rates of anorexics than non-identical twins.[3] There are currently international studies examining this area.[4]

Anecdotal evidence has reported that the families of anorexic girls show certain dysfunctional characteristics. These families tend to be:

- conflict avoidant
- over-enmeshed

- over-protective
- rigid.

Where there is conflict between parents, the anorexic frequently finds herself involved. Certain theorists go so far as to propose that the illness serves to *deflect* attention from the parental conflict.[5]

Psychological theories stress that anorexics tend to be perfectionists with poor self-esteem. This is a difficult personality combination. Anorexics tend to judge their success or failure in life on *measurable* achievements; such as weight loss and academic performance.[6] They do not measure their worth in abstract concepts such as kindness or generosity: rather, they congratulate themselves on how much weight has been lost or how little was eaten at dinner.

Another psychological theory is that anorexic girls do not want to grow up into independent, sexually mature women.[7] Of course, this is an 'unconscious' decision. The thinner they become, the more their puberty slows down until they ultimately stop menstruating.

According to the diagnostic criteria, anorexics cannot lose the intense fear of gaining weight. Even if they are underweight, they dread becoming obese. They refuse to maintain their weight at a healthy level. In addition to this fear of fat, they have a markedly disturbed body image. They see themselves as fat even when their weight is below average and to everyone else they appear underweight.[8] More rarely, they express hatred of their bodies and overestimate the size of their body parts such as thighs or bottoms. Anorexics tend to deny the problem and have very limited insight. They are often depressed or even suicidal.

Numerous neurotransmitters are implicated in anorexia, although the details remain very complex and obscure. To mention but two neurotransmitters: high opiate levels promote fasting, as do high serotonin levels. Certain opiates are raised in anorexia while others are decreased.[9]

DR DORA: Starvation leads to food obsessions

In anorexia, there is an ambivalent relationship with food. On the one hand, anorexics restrict what they eat to the point of starvation. Yet, they also seem obsessed by food. They develop peculiar rituals with their food: they may cut it into very small pieces, move it around on the plate or eat it very slowly. When food is not being eaten, they may hoard it, hide it or carry it in their pockets. They tend to use all sorts of condiments with their food to drown the taste completely. Food becomes a preoccupation: they may collect recipes, cook for the family or choose jobs involving catering. Apart from with food, they are obsessive in many other areas, such as weighing themselves on the scale *repeatedly*.

This eccentric behaviour around food is remarkably similar to what has been observed with starving prisoners of war.[10] In fact, some researchers propose that anorexics are starving and starvation causes the bizarre behaviour.

In the 1950s, some research was done with normal male volunteers who agreed to be starved in an experiment. Soon, these men developed an overwhelming preoccupation with food. Even their dreams centred on eating. They stole food and hoarded it. If given an opportunity, they would binge and sometimes purge. As far as their emotions were concerned, they showed changes characteristic of anorexia nervosa: they got depressed, had poor concentration, withdrew socially and had poor libido. These previously well-balanced men became completely obsessive and their outside interests narrowed down completely.[11]

In addition to being depressed, anorexics suffer from other psychiatric problems. About 10% of them also have an anxiety disorder called obsessive compulsive disorder. People suffering from this condition have intrusive, recurrent 'obsessive' thoughts that cause them severe anxiety and/or compulsive ritualistic behaviours that alleviate anxiety (see DSM IV).

DR DORA: How the body is affected by starvation

A starving body faces many dangers.

- As anorexics become 'skin and bone', they lose their fat stores. Body fat is essential for oestrogen synthesis. Many anorexics cannot maintain oestrogen production; so menstruation stops and their bones become brittle. But the relationship between oestrogen and body fat is complex. In some cases, menstruation may stop before weight loss is severe. In recovering anorexics, menstrual periods may remain irregular for many months even though weight is gained.[12]
- Anorexics may eventually lose their secondary sexual characteristics, becoming flat chested with sparse pubic hair and no curves.
- Blood pressure drops and the heartbeat may become irregular, abnormally slow or fast.
- They always feel cold owing to their poor circulation and inadequate temperature control.
- They have many gastrointestinal complaints including constipation, bloating and abdominal pain.
- In severe cases, dehydration and epileptic fits may occur.
- They may become anaemic with low haemoglobin, white cells and platelets.

Some anorexics eventually die of starvation.

One of two things can happen now: the dysfunctional eater will simply take measures of control even further; or she can lose control and give in to her hunger out of complete exhaustion and desperation. Once she has given in, she starts on the journey of bulimia nervosa, which, to a large extent, mimics the activity of a drug addiction.

This is what Ann does. She gives in to the enormous urge to eat. Because she has denied this urge for so long it has become powerful;

all encompassing. This is an age-old survival instinct largely governed subconsciously by serotonin, or the lack of serotonin.

By this time she has built up such a feeling of self-loathing and guilt that the ensuing submission to food is an act of both catharsis and self-punishment – proving to herself that her body is truly weak and gluttonous, deserving of nothing besides being fat. And so the binge begins.

It is no coincidence that the foods chosen are of two types, often satisfying both criteria at once:

- Quick-releasing carbohydrates.
- 'Nursery foods': foods that not only remind the eater of childhood and its associated happy memories, but that are also quick and easy to eat, filling the gap with little or no effort.

The choice of fast-releasing carbohydrates is to stimulate a massive surge of the brain's calming chemical (serotonin) – a much-needed substance after such a long period of deprivation. Nursery foods are chosen because they provide a feeling of safety.

This is where, I believe, the urge to be a little girl again comes in. The dieter is often a young woman, struggling to cope with impending womanhood and its responsibilities, but challenging this even further. She is nervous enough at the prospect of entering womanhood with all of its uncertainties and exciting promises, but with her lack of eating, these emotions are further compounded physically, by the diminishing serotonin production and its resultant symptoms. The feeling of being out of control whilst fighting her body serves to confirm her belief that she cannot cope with adulthood. So, she attempts control by controlling the one thing she has personal control over: food. This calorie deprivation further decreases the production of serotonin, which also serves to intensify the depressive symptoms. Thus, the psychiatric depression she feels drives the nail even further into her self-doubt, and proves her insecurities that she cannot cope as an adult, as she knows she is expected to, very soon.

For this reason Ann secretly chooses to submit to her child-like needs to eat and feel satisfied. The submission shames her though – it conflicts with her perception of control. She believes that her childhood (and the relaxed, responsive and fulfilling eating patterns that are synonymous with childhood) must be shunned. Yet she secretly chooses foods that she enjoyed as a child;

food that conjures up a time when she was not expected to make any decisions or behave with adult responsibility; a time when everything was done for her and no one was disappointed by her lack of control.

Because she feels that she has failed herself and everyone's expectations of her as a young woman capable of exercising self-control, it will make no difference whether she eats a little or a lot. As she starts eating, she feels a sublime rush caused by the feel-good serotonin flooding her brain. The feeling is pure bliss; it is impossible to stop now.

Consequently, she eats, and eats some more, and yet more. Desperately she attempts to taste as many flavours possible, all at once. To prolong the feeling, she swallows quickly, not chewing properly. An exquisite feeling of happiness engulfs her. She feels contented, sleepy, and wonderful – the same way she remembers feeling as a little child. This is what she has missed – the uncomplicated life of childhood. If only she could feel, and be allowed to feel like this all the time.

But she knows it is impossible. Firstly, ladies do not eat like this, and secondly, it will make her fat. Even small amounts of food make her fat, she reasons: the evidence shows clearly on her waist!

Flooded by self-hatred, Ann looks at the mess before her. She has consumed a shocking amount of food. Her worst fears are confirmed: her body has no control whatsoever, unlike everyone else's. She would never be worthy of being called an adult. Adults are disciplined. They have the ability to say no, and to stop. Mortally disappointed, she realises that she could never be that strong. The scene before her eyes bears silent proof.

Then her stomach lurches at the sight. Only one thing to do now. Quickly she runs to the toilet and immediately purges the food, thinking that she does not deserve the feelings of satisfaction brought on by the food. She simply cannot behave like a child!

Relieved to be free of the food again, she contemplates her actions. The food can't harm her now, she thinks. It tried to 'get at' her, but she prevented any damage by purging quickly enough. But the event has left her feeling sick and exhausted, and with a splitting headache. Moreover, she feels angry with herself for allowing things to get out of hand, and guilty because she enjoyed the food so much. An overwhelming need to sleep engulfs her, to make it all go away... to escape this horrible adult existence that she cannot cope with, and never will... and to dream herself into another place ... where things are happy, warm and calm ...

The above is a typical example of binge eating and the resultant violent fluctuation of blood sugar levels, and therefore serotonin. As she eats quickly and uncontrollably, driven by powerful instincts (the intensity of which often depends on how prolonged and severe the restrictive period has been) her serotonin levels increase, calming her, making her feel good and relaxed.

The intensity of this experience is also a matter of starting point. If she was feeling very low, then even a small change in brain chemicals will cause her to feel euphoric by comparison. Following the euphoria, her conscious thought re-introduces guilt and anxiety. What had been a pleasurable experience now fills her with despair as she recalls her lack of control. Furthermore, she reminds herself that, in essence, she is unworthy to experience pleasure.

After the purging (an exhausting process in itself), her blood sugar levels plummet. The consequent hypoglycaemia brings a decrease in serotonin levels, thus inducing the depressive feelings and symptoms. Sleeping is a means of escape, and is also a natural shock-reaction after the purging.

When she wakes up her blood sugar levels will remain low, and her need for more carbohydrate foods will again be overwhelming. She will then enter the new cycle of avoidance and excessive control, followed by a peak of despair. Following this course she will again lose control, binge, experience the serotonin high, and then purge, with the serotonin levels falling again.

It is obvious how this cycle follows that of the drug addict. Each period of restriction only serves to increase the need for food and intensifies the physiological need for eating. The resultant binge often feels as though it should be bigger than the previous one in order to reach the same 'high', because each time the baseline is that much lower. When the high is reached, however, anxiety increases with every guilty mouthful. She feels the pleasure her body experiences by being 'out of control', and she hates it. The anorexic's fears of being weak / out of control are confirmed when she purges after the binge. She feels yet more inadequate and undeserving of any joy. With each binge her self-confidence decreases and purging becomes the only way to remove the physical joy her body experiences by eating. In this way she becomes more dependent on the purge itself.

DR DORA: What is bulimia nervosa?

While the phenomenon of voluntary starvation (anorexia nervosa) has been recognised for centuries, it was only in the 1970s that reports began emerging of uncontrolled eating in normal weight individuals. Bulimia nervosa was first described as a clinical entity in 1979, and was given its name. There is much overlap between anorexia nervosa and bulimia nervosa and many sufferers have features of both conditions. An example of this overlap is that an anorexic may 'evolve' over time to develop bingeing and purging behaviour.[13] Almost half of all anorexics eventually show bulimic behaviour and up to 80% of bulimics have a history of anorexia.

Bulimics are diagnosed according to the following criteria (see DSM IV):

- They have recurrent episodes of *binge eating* where they consume huge amounts of food within a short time (two hours).
- During the binge, they feel out of control, guilty and disgusting.
- After a binge, they show *compensatory behaviour* such as vomiting, fasting, purging by using laxatives or diuretics, or excessive exercising.
- This cycle has to occur at least twice a week for a period of three months to make the diagnosis.
- Bulimics tend to evaluate themselves in terms of their body shape, weight and size.

How common is bulimia?

Initially, it was believed that bulimia is very rare. It took an early eating disorders researcher over six years to collect just 30 cases![14] However, now we know that bulimia is more common than anorexia. Researchers and medical practitioners simply don't detect it. If the sufferer is of normal weight, it can remain a secret disorder for years. It affects between 1% and 3% of young women.[15] It is up to 50 times more common in females than in males. The onset of bulimia is in adolescence or in the early twenties, which is later than the onset of anorexia.

If one moves away from the strict diagnostic criteria of bulimia nervosa mentioned above, it appears that occasional episodes of bingeing and purging are very common in young women. One study of female students at an American university showed that 40% displayed bulimic-type behaviour.

A binge in detail ...

Binges are often triggered by an unpleasant event. Various mood states such as depression, boredom, loneliness or anxiety may also precipitate a binge. They tend to occur in secret or at night. High calorie, sweet, soft food is consumed in vast quantities. There is such urgency about a binge that food may not be chewed and little attention is paid to its taste or texture. During the binge, a bulimic does not experience satiety. The binge comes to an end because of a painfully distended abdomen, bloating, physical exhaustion or the arrival of another person. After the binge, there is a feeling of drowsiness, depression and self-disgust. This has been called post-binge anguish.

Vomiting frequently follows a binge and can be self-induced. It relieves the feeling of abdominal distension and allows the binge to occur without weight gain. Many bulimics experience a lifting of mood after vomiting.

DR DORA: What causes bulimia?

We do not know the answer to this question but there are many theories about the cause of bulimia. As usual in psychiatry, they can be divided into biological, social and psychological factors.

Biologically:

- Several neurotransmitters have been implicated in bulimia: specifically serotonin, noradrenalin and the opiates. Serotonin levels are typically low in bulimia.[16] Remember tryptophan, the amino acid precursor of serotonin? Well, cutting out dietary tryptophan has more dramatic effects in bulimics than in normal women. A study of the role of serotonin in bulimia found that after being deprived of dietary tryptophan, bulimic women showed worse depression, mood swings and desire to binge than normal women. This suggests that in bulimics, the brain serotonergic system is more vulnerable to diet than in normal women. [17]

- Noradrenalin levels are also low in bulimia. [18] This may explain the high incidence of depression, low blood pressure and slow heart rate found in bulimics. Starvation and intermittent dieting lower noradrenalin levels. Just to complicate matters, in other brain areas, noradrenalin levels are high. This is believed to be responsible for bingeing. [19]

- The blood levels of endorphins (opiates) are raised in some bulimics.[20] We know that endorphin levels increase after vomiting in normal individuals. Perhaps bulimics become 'addicted' to the mood lift experienced after vomiting, which is caused by high circulating endorphins?

- Hormones that control appetite and feeding behaviour are also identified as potentially responsible for bulimia.[21, 22] One of these hormones, peptide YY, stimulates feeding. It is found at abnormally high levels in bulimics. Some researchers propose that high levels of this hormone drive the uncontrollable bingeing behaviour seen in bulimics. [23] A digestive hormone called cholecystokinin, which has the opposite effect (it *decreases* appetite), is believed to be faulty in bulimia. [24]

- Another interesting finding is that the vomiting centre of the brain is situated close to the emotional centre (the limbic system). This may explain the connection between a mood state and the action of vomiting.

- Genetic factors may also play a role in bulimia. Frequently, there is a family history of eating disorders, depression, alcohol abuse or obesity.[25]

At this point, it remains unclear whether the biological factors mentioned above are the result or the cause of the eating disorder. Much more research is needed to clarify the issue of causality.

Socially:

- In terms of their social experience, bulimics have often been physically or sexually abused in childhood. They may have experienced early loss or bereavement.

- Society's emphasis on thinness has been alluded to in the discussion of anorexia. Perhaps it is due to this pressure that bulimics start dieting. When they 'slip up' on a forbidden food, they react by eating even more. This may escalate into a binge.

Psychologically:

- Binges may be triggered by stress, arguments, disappointment or frustration.
- Overeating may present an opportunity for the bulimic to experience some control in her life. She learns to use bingeing and vomiting as a method to alleviate frustration. However, the relief is short-lived. No sooner than the binge occurs, guilt and a worsening of depression follow.

The physical dangers of bulimia
It is difficult for a family member to recognise a bulimic as the signs are often subtle. However, bulimics do undergo some physical changes. While these are less dramatic than in anorexia, bulimia can be life threatening.

Bingeing is responsible for several problems:

- Bulimics may develop a painless swelling of the large salivary glands in their lower cheeks (the parotid glands). When these are enlarged, they lead to a 'hamster looking' face.
- Following a huge binge, there is danger that the stomach may rupture.
- Many bulimics report irregular menstrual cycles.

Vomiting and purging cause different complications.

- Vomiting disturbs the levels of blood electrolytes. These chemicals are essential to life even though they are present in tiny amounts. Low potassium levels cause muscle weakness and pain, skin numbness and irregular heart beat. In extreme cases, kidney damage and epilepsy may result.
- When dental enamel comes into contact with gastric acid during vomiting, it may become eroded. This leads to caries, fillings and tooth loss.
- Swelling of the extremities may occur. To counteract this, many eating disordered individuals take diuretics (medications that promote water loss through urinating). However, when the body becomes dehydrated, it automatically retains more fluid, so that the end result is *weight gain*, not weight loss. Unscrupulous diuretic use can be extremely dangerous.
- Constipation, stomach ulcers and oesophageal bleeding may also occur.
- The voice may become chronically hoarse.
- Calluses may develop on the knuckles of those who induce vomiting.

This destructive cycle is a serotonin roller coaster, and it can be stopped IMMEDIATELY. The effects of severe calorie cutting on the mind are devastating, as the example above clearly illustrates. It can be equally damaging to the body. Before we examine the way the body is affected by dieting, let's quickly recap on metabolism.

10 HOW DIETING AFFECTS YOUR METABOLISM

If you haven't read **The X Diet** yet, here is some background on metabolism to put you in the picture (without all the baffling medical jargon – it is important that you discover and understand all the facts clearly).

The body has an intricate and elegant mechanism of controlling the amount of fat it carries. In many people, however, this mechanism malfunctions for various reasons. But for now, let's only consider the way it is supposed to function.

Leptin

Fat cells produce a chemical substance called leptin, a 'messenger' which notifies the body of its fat status (i.e. how much fat is present at any time). As the body grows fatter, the expanding fat cells produce more leptin. The leptin serves to control the amount of fat on the body by unconsciously signalling the hypothalamus (again!) to:

- increase the amount of energy burned up (metabolism speeds up), and
- decrease the appetite (eat less),
- with the result that the fat cells are burned up, and diminish again in size.

Not only does leptin serve to keep the body slim (by monitoring the size of the fat cells), but it also has a memory, perhaps to keep fat cells big for storage, if it has memorised a previously experienced famine situation.

Leptin resistance

To date, researchers have found many biological reasons for obesity, none of which include gluttony! Leptin dysfunctions are the main cause of obesity, but what is quite frightening, is that one type of leptin dysfunction can actually be induced by calorie restriction. This is called leptin resistance, but before we discuss that, let's first look at some other leptin abnormalities:

Why do some people get fat?

The following are reasons why some people get fat:

No leptin production

The fat cells are unable to produce leptin and the body has absolutely no way of knowing that it is getting fatter – it receives no signals to increase the metabolism and decrease the appetite. Although this has been documented in three people in the world it is extremely rare.

Too little leptin

The fat cells do produce leptin, but in amounts far less than required to fully convey the signals. As the body gains fat, it only receives partial signals.

Faulty leptin

The fat cells produce correct amounts of leptin but it is faulty (i.e. odd-shaped). This odd shape prevents the signals (that fat is being gained) from reaching the body.

Faulty leptin 'ears'

The fat cells produce leptin in normal amounts and shape, but the leptin 'ears' of the brain are faulty. Though the signals reach the brain, it is 'deaf' to the signals. Again the body gets fatter, unnoticed.

Too few leptin 'ears'

The fat cells produce leptin in perfect amounts and shape, but there are not enough leptin 'ears' (or receptors) in the brain to fully register the amount of leptin trying to get their signals across.

For instance, to bring the concept down to easy numbers to understand, say the brain should have 100 open 'ears') listening for leptin signals. If the fat cells produce five leptins, then only five of the 'ears' are needed to listen, because the body has only got a little fatter. But the other 95 'ears' are still idle, waiting for a possible future signal. If the body gets very fat, chances are that 90 leptins are produced, thus notifying 90 'ears' that there is a large amount of fat present, and that action is required and appetite must be decreased dramatically.

However, in some people there may be only, say, 10 leptin 'ears' ever open. The rest are not idle, waiting for a response – they are blocked. The body is safe if it only gets a little fatter (to produce five extra leptins because five 'ears' can hear this), but if it gets very fat, and say, 100 leptins are produced, this spells trouble. The hypothalamus only has 'ears' open for five leptins; and it is unable to hear the other 95. This is called being 'leptin resistant'. The hypothalamus is deaf or resistant to the amounts of leptin being produced, and while it gets fatter and fatter, it remains under the impression that it is only a little bit fatter. Adequate adjustment can therefore not be made and the fat cells increase unchecked.

Self-induced leptin resistance

The leptin process and all the leptin 'ears' in the brain function normally until you embark on a strict calorie-cutting diet. Through a long and complex cascade of events during decreased calorie intake, the fully functional leptin 'ears', are instructed to block themselves to the leptin signal because the body has entered a famine (it does not realise the famine is self-inflicted!) This is so that fat can be accumulated (if eaten). Consequently, a beautifully healthy and normally-controlled body begins its starving descent into self-induced leptin resistance. The leptin 'ears' (or receptors) have been down-regulated ('or blocked up') into leptin resistance.

The process of self-induced leptin resistance can be summarised as follows:

When starved, the body realises that it is going through a famine and so stores this information into its memory. This body, so beautifully adaptable, now reprogrammes its whole metabolic process to be able to store more fat in the fat cells in preparation for another period of famine. In this way the body prepares itself so that these accumulated fat stores can be used for energy when such a famine occurs – an unbelievably brilliant and effective survival technique.

By the way, once this adaptation has occurred the only way the new, fat-accumulating body can possibly lose this newly acquired fat stores is by starving itself. This is why each attempt at cutting calories will only be effective if less and less is eaten with every diet. And, as you may have noticed, the body will silently and continuously reprogramme itself each and every time you go on a severely calorie-restricted diet, thus turning it into a more effective fat storing machine with every subsequent diet. What's more, once the fat has been forced to be burnt up by starvation, this new body composition can only be maintained if next to nothing is eaten for the rest of time.

Looking at it from a physiologist's point of view, one has to marvel at the intricacies and perfect balance our wonderful bodies have for smooth survival and realise that this 'squirrelling' of fat stores is precisely one of the main reasons mankind is still on this earth after thousands of years of famines and droughts.

On the other hand, I hope it has given you enough of an eye-opener into the dangers of calorie cutting and the life-changing consequences. This is why it has been proven that the more you calorie-cut to lose weight, the more you are setting yourself up to be a fatter person in the future.

Sound hopeless? Fortunately not! And there are ways to get the metabolic rate back to normal; one being clearly never to calorie-cut again unless you enjoy being a food-obsessed, starving, defensive and perpetually uptight waif whose narcissism makes others feel you really aren't much fun to be around. (Does this sound familiar at all?)

Insulin and blood sugar

Now that the complexities of leptin function (and dysfunction) are clear, let's progress to something that can be measured and control-led: insulin and blood sugar. You are probably a bit at a loss now, but let me explain. It may sound extremely complicated at first, but read on carefully. The better you understand leptin and insulin, the clearer it will be how you can actually rectify this devastating situation you may have been born with, or else have dieted your body into.

When you eat carbohydrates (bread, potatoes, pasta, rice and so on), they dissolve into their component sugars, which you need for energy (remember high school biology?) Carbohydrates not only taste wonderful; they also keep you alive (the tastebuds have been telling the body this for millennia). Yes, quite simply, although 'man cannot live on bread alone', it will certainly form a damn good staple while he searches for the balance!

When the blood sugar stores dwindle, the body sends a hunger signal calling for replenishment. As you eat carbohydrates, they dissolve into sugar. The sugar floods and concentrates in the blood resulting in a sublime feeling of happiness and immediately improving general well-being (remember serotonin production?). These miraculous sets of events continue without us even being aware, delivering energy to our muscles, keeping the body happily and healthily in perfect equilibrium.

When the blood becomes filled with sugar (you have just eaten a carbohydrate, for example a potato), the pancreas releases a whole force of 'storage policemen', called insulin, to deliver this energy to the required places in the body, such as the muscles. The active insulin swims through this very sugary blood, and to clear the blood again, directs the sugar towards the muscles all over the body. Upon reaching the entrance to each of the muscles, the insulin pushes on the insulin 'doors' of the various muscles and forces the sugar through them so as to store the sugar in the muscles.

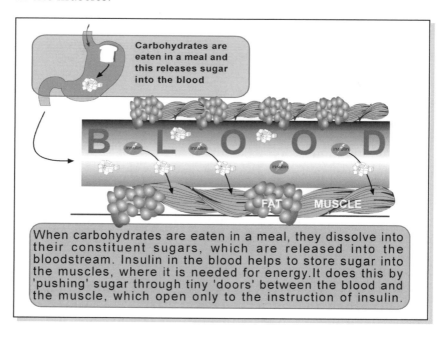

Carbohydrates are eaten in a meal and this releases sugar into the blood

When carbohydrates are eaten in a meal, they dissolve into their constituent sugars, which are released into the bloodstream. Insulin in the blood helps to store sugar into the muscles, where it is needed for energy. It does this by 'pushing' sugar through tiny 'doors' between the blood and the muscle, which open only to the instruction of insulin.

Once the insulin has completed its job (storing the sugar), it goes 'off duty'. Now the blood contains a normal, steady flow of sugar again – just enough to keep things running as usual.

In fact, a steady flow of sugar in the blood at all times is vital to staying alive. Sugar is therefore not the evil substance it is made out to be!

Insulin resistance

Returning to the insulin, it is released in amounts corresponding to the amount of sugar in the blood (the blood sugar level), which in turn depends on the type of carbohydrates eaten. You will remember that some carbohydrates dissolve into sugar very quickly (high GI), thus requiring a large amount of insulin to store the sudden, huge sugar load. Some carbohydrates, however, dissolve much more slowly (low GI) thus necessitating a considerably smaller amount of insulin to be released.

This is exactly where leptin problems show up!

You see, leptin 'ears' and insulin 'doors' communicate 24 hours a day. This doesn't warrant any excitement, unless the leptin 'ears' begin blocking themselves up (remember, down-regulation from calorie cutting). At this point, the insulin 'doors' copy this 'blocking-up' mechanism, and do the same. Yes, the insulin doors lock themselves up.

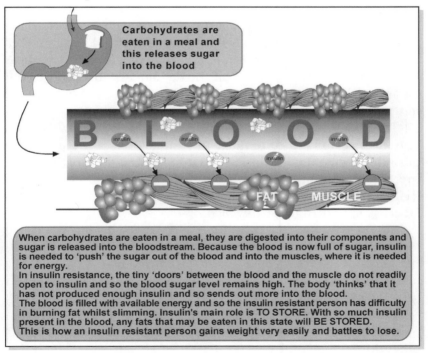

Carbohydrates are eaten in a meal and this releases sugar into the blood

When carbohydrates are eaten in a meal, they are digested into their components and sugar is released into the bloodstream. Because the blood is now full of sugar, insulin is needed to 'push' the sugar out of the blood and into the muscles, where it is needed for energy.
In insulin resistance, the tiny 'doors' between the blood and the muscle do not readily open to insulin and so the blood sugar level remains high. The body 'thinks' that it has not produced enough insulin and so sends out more into the blood.
The blood is filled with available energy and so the insulin resistant person has difficulty in burning fat whilst slimming. Insulin's main role is TO STORE. With so much insulin present in the blood, any fats that may be eaten in this state will BE STORED.
This is how an insulin resistant person gains weight very easily and battles to lose.

Consequently, when sugar is rapidly released into the blood (you have just eaten a high GI carbohydrate), the sugar level rises dramatically, and lots of insulin is released, ready to store the sugar into the muscles. But now the insulin doors to the muscles have locked themselves up, leaving only a few doors open for insulin to store the sugar. Consequently it takes much, much longer to push all of this excess sugar into the muscles, and the blood sugar level remain high for a long time. This is called insulin resistance.

'So what?' you ask.

Well, since sugar is the body's fuel, the blood must be the fuel tank, holding the sugar until it is pushed into the muscles, right? So, if your fuel tank is full for a long time (the sugar level stays high because insulin cannot work effectively), then there is plenty of fuel to use when needed. With so much available energy being present in the blood, the reserve tank (fat storage) isn't used for energy. Therefore, you stay fat and furthermore, battle to lose that fat, despite dieting.

Let's recap on this. Your blood (fuel tank) is normally at a low fuel content (sugar level), just enough to keep you functioning normally. Because the content of your fuel tank is fairly low, it will regularly 'dip into' the reserve tank (fat cells) for energy. This means that small amounts of fat are continuously being burned when the blood sugar level is normal. Then comes the entry of a sugar flood (a carbohydrate meal), and the fuel tank fills to capacity (the sugar level rises high). This means that the fuel tank is full, and will not dip into the reserve tank (it has no need to – there is so much sugar in the blood).

This cessation of fat usage while sugar levels are high should only happen for the 20 minutes or so that it takes the insulin to push the sugar out of the blood and into the muscles. So, this interruption of fat burning really is of no consequence, because before long, the insulin removes all the excess sugar from the blood, and fat cells are burned for energy again.

But, in Syndrome X, or insulin resistance, the insulin 'doors' are locked up and the insulin cannot do its job effectively. As a result, the sugar level stays high for a more prolonged period. Because the fuel tank remains filled to capacity for a long time, fat burning ceases for a long time, too.

What's more, if the sugar level is high there will be lots of insulin present, trying to store sugars, albeit unsuccessfully. It also stores other things, including fats, if eaten. So, if you are an insulin resistant person whose sugar levels stay high, then the subsequent increase in insulin will deal with any fat included in the meal that is now floating in the blood by very promptly storing it in your fat cells.

Thus, someone without insulin resistance can include fats in their diet, and most of them will be burned up effectively. The insulin-resistant person, however, will be that storage machine we spoke of earlier, immediately storing every tiny bit of fat eaten, including hidden fats!

This is exactly why leptin and insulin communicate as they do – to make sure that when the body is subjected to a famine, it is geared up perfectly to store fat very quickly, in case the famine hits again.

Now you know why some people get fat very quickly, and why some people don't. It is not quite a matter of eating too much, is it? I hope that as more people understand how complex weight gain is and how dangerous rapid weight loss can be, they will consult with medical and dietetics practitioners to find a solution rather than repeatedly calorie-restricting themselves towards permanent insulin resistance (otherwise known as diabetes).

You should now have a clear understanding of why calorie restricting can make you fat. Read on, and discover some more horrifying truths about how calorie restriction can affect your body. Not only can calorie restriction be linked to clinical depression and chronic mental illness. In addition, it can catalyse the descent into grave lifestyle disorders, associated with insulin resistance.

But this is not the only reason the metabolism slows down. First understand all of the reasons, and then your eyes will open to the fact that we have a global epidemic on our hands.

How dieting affects your body

I take poetic licence when I assume the subject of this book to be a woman. I do see many, many more women with eating problems than men, but so does an oncologist see many more female breast cancer patients than male. Neither conditions, however, are gender-specific. I wish to make it clear that I address both men and women in this chapter, using the feminine person as a subject.

To lose weight you always cut down on the amount of food you eat. You cut your consumption in half; or measure it against something; or weigh it out to less than you want; or call it a substantially scientific-sounding name but drink cabbage soup for weeks. Whichever way you look at it, you are cutting calories. This is because you apply simple laws of physics to your body: if you don't put in as much as you expend you will get smaller. Right?

Wrong!

You are *what* you eat

Your body is not a simple seesaw of energy balance. You are not a product of how much you eat at all. No matter how many people keep telling you that. If this was the case then we'd all be gigantic masses of blubber with a brain. You are what you eat, not how much you eat! The example below clearly illustrates my point:

Let's pretend your metabolism is measured as being 2000 Cal/day. This means that on average, without exercise, your body routinely burns up 2000 calories of energy each day, just by living (breathing, pumping your heart, etc).

You calculate that you probably eat 2000 Cal/day of food. If you continued eating exactly the same way, but added a chocolate each afternoon, which added exactly 500 Cal/day to your input, then you would gain 36kg of fat in a year. This is clearly impossible; otherwise very few people would be able to walk after six years. Your body starts adapting to this new input, and auto-adjusts its metabolism to match it. Some of this auto-adjustment means to take the fat from the chocolate and add it to the body. This increases the total weight carried around, thereby increasing the output. But the increase in energy intake causes the body to start burning a little more energy each day, so that eventually your daily output becomes 2500 Cal/day.

Does this mean that obese people have a very high metabolic rate? Yes, absolutely! This is one of the least understood facts about obesity. Someone who is very overweight – 200kg, for example – has a much bigger job to do, carrying that extra weight around. (Think of a person who weighs 70kg, who carries another two persons on his or her back.) This is obviously an enormous amount of energy expended, and, in fact, most of us would be too weak to do it.

However the obese do it all the time. They cannot 'take it off' and walk faster, for instance. So, to cope, their bodies have become much stronger: they have built much more muscle to carry this load. Because muscle is what burns energy in the body, the obese body burns much more energy at any one time than a thin person does.

'Why then do they stay fat?' you ask. Because their auto-regulation system is either genetically faulty or it has been damaged by too much yo-yo dieting, or it is insulin resistant. But if it were as simple as energy-in/energy-out there would be no fat people in the world, would there?

If your body is not a simple seesaw of energy, then why do you gain or lose weight?

Your 'reserve tank'

Not all calories are equal. This is rule number one. Calories from carbohydrates do very different things to your body than do calories from fats, for example. And that is why you need a balanced diet, so that the different parts of different foods can do different jobs in your body.

Carbohydrates are your body's 'fuel', as it were. Carbohydrates release sugar into the blood stream, and this sugar is the main source of energy. Energy for thinking, breathing, digesting, walking, laughing, sleeping, etc. And, just like a car, the body needs fuel every so often; otherwise it has to dip into the reserve tank for extra fuel. Now, the reserve tank should only be used for emergencies, right? Well, the same applies to your body. You have a 'reserve tank' to store energy and for use in emergencies (famine and drought).

Your reserve tank is made up of:

- **Stored carbohydrates** (but this is only a tiny amount, in the liver and muscles. The body cannot store carbohydrates well at all.)
- **Fat** visibly stored in the gut, thighs, arms, etc. as well as hidden, surrounding the heart, kidneys, and liver, to keep them safe and warm.
- **Protein**, which is what makes up the obvious leg and arm muscles, as well as the heart, stomach and gastrointestinal tract, uterus, liver, kidneys etc. – in fact, everything that is precious to your make-up.

The biggest (and least attractive) part of this reserve tank is fat. And this is usually what needs to be used up, somehow. You may well ask whether it is logical then to never fill up your fuel tank, so that your body runs on empty the whole time; running completely from energy from fat? Well, this does work to a certain extent. Starvation will always make you lose weight. (But so will chopping off your right arm. Very quick, very successful, because you weigh less.) But what happens then? Well, you get fat again, In fact, when you cut calories and rapidly lose weight you will usually get fat again even more quickly – and even fatter than before the crash-course in self-deprivation.

This is because when you calorie-cut, your body is forced to use up only the reserve tank. Remember that this reserve tank is largely fat, but it also is made up of proteins from your muscles. In fact, the less you eat, the deeper into the reserve tank your body has to dip, in order to keep you alive! You see, fat is burned to yield energy, but it can only burn very slowly, yielding tiny amounts of energy at a time. If the reserve tank is all that is being burned, then fat and protein must burn to yield enough energy to keep going.

For example, you may have a metabolic output of 2000 Cal/day (the amount you burn up) and you decide to eat half of everything, which is 1000 Cal/day. This is not a lot of fuel at all and therefore your tank runs out very quickly during the day and starts dipping into the reserve tank. You lose fat. Fantastic! But you have forgotten the other bit of fuel that makes up the reserve tank: Protein.

Therefore you lose fat and muscle.

'So what?' you may say, 'I'm thin, and that is all that matters!' Well that can seem all that matters, until the next few weeks of eating 'normally' again start turning you into the Michelin Man.

This happens because you lost muscle when your body was forced to draw from the reserve tank only, and muscle burns energy fairly quickly. Your metabolism is mainly dependent on how much muscle you have. The more muscle you have, the more energy your body will burn up each day. But, the less muscle you have, the less energy you will burn up each day. Simple.

By eating half the calories, your body kept going by dipping deeply into your reserve tank. Your body had to use up muscle mass, and so its ability to burn calories (your metabolism) decreased to 1000 Cal/day.

If you then eat any more than 1000 Cal/day, especially if it is fat, it will be stored as fat, because your body can no longer burn energy as quickly. Your metabolism has auto-regulated itself to expend the same number of calories as you have been putting in! Which is now much less than before!

Because you indicated to your body that 1000 Cal/day was all that was available to eat, it decreased its energy use to accommodate this decreased amount. If it didn't do this, and carried on with a high rate of energy use, you would deplete your energy stores and die very quickly! Clever, don't you think? For this reason the weight loss is dramatic: but only about half of the weight lost is fat. The rest is muscle!

This process of auto-cannibalisation (i.e. using the muscle mass) means literally eating one's self away, in order to survive through this barbaric starvation phase.

The body has learned to do this on purpose because humans are moving creatures, thus requiring our energy stores to move with us. Plants, by virtue of being firmly rooted to the ground, have their food supply (the earth) right there whenever it is required.

But humans are not planted anywhere! We move away from our food source most of the time. And so, the more we move away from this food source, the bigger our portable storage compartment needs to be.

If you were a human being who always ate on the hour, you would be 're-fuelling' every hour. You would never dip into your reserve tank, and so your reserve tank would not need to be that big, would it?

If, however, you were a human being who moved away from your food source for the whole day, each day, then your body would be forced to dip into your reserve tank a lot, wouldn't it? So, you would use up all the fat and some of the muscle to auto-regulate the metabolism down to the limited number of calories put in. However each evening, at supper, you would fill up your reserve tank first and then the rest of the petrol tank.

This reserve tank keeps being depleted every day, and is now ready for you to fill it up with more fat, for the next day. So, your body quickly replaces all of the lost fat from that day, for the next day's long journey away from food.

What's more, the human body has the unique ability to be able to change the size of that reserve tank. It can be 'programmed' in this way fairly easily, to respond to how far from food you may take yourself each day. The longer you leave between meals, the bigger your reserve tank must be in order to keep you alive!

It's very simple, really. The less you eat, the more your body auto-regulates itself to using up less energy. And the less often you eat the bigger your storage capacity needs to be.

So, by eating less, and skipping meals, you are in essence telling your body that from now on it will encounter less food, and less often. So, your clever body simply adapts with no problem to having bigger storage space (bigger fat stores), and reducing the energy used up (eating away your muscle mass so that your metabolism is lower). This way, it ensures that you carry enough fat around to keep you alive for even longer than you have already challenged it to. Furthermore, it ensures that you get so sluggish, that no matter how far you go from your food source, you will not use up that much energy each day, anyway.

Perfect adaptation for bush-survival, isn't it? But you can see where it all goes wrong in your quest for thinness, each time you calorie-cut: you are just telling your body to become increasingly efficient at 'storing' because you keep going through a famine, over and over again!

We need to understand our bodies in the 'animal' context because this is how our hormonal structure was formed thousands of years ago. We humans have only very recently started purposefully starving ourselves at will. And our bodies simply don't understand why we keep going through so many famines and droughts. So, the body just keeps on, miraculously, keeping us alive, and ensuring that we are well stocked for the next famine. And it does this by re-setting all of our hormones, and adjusting nearly every functioning part of our bodies, in careful protection of our being. One of these adjustments is to our serotonin functioning, as we have learned.

The less carbohydrates we ingest, the less serotonin production is stimulated. And the less we feel at peace with ourselves.

So, calorie cutting simply is not successful in the long term. Instead we turn our bodies into storage machines, and our brains into obsessive and unhappy masses of anxiety. And it's not as simple as just trying to be 'normal' again, or attempting to return to moderation, because we have successfully disrupted all 'normal' and 'moderate' physical equilibrium.

Now, read on, and be educated.

Carbohydrates cannot make you fat

If you eat excessive carbohydrates, the biological pathway can lead to increased fat storage. But, if you eat fat-free, the amount of carbohydrates you would need to eat in order to fulfil this 'excessive' capacity is not humanly possible. So relax, eat fat free, and you will not be able to make fat from carbohydrates!

Carbohydrates cannot make you fat. They can only keep your metabolism normal and return your brain to normal, controlled thinking patterns. After all, we don't call it 'grey matter' for nothing.

11 THE DIETING MENTALITY – A FORM OF DEPRESSION?

The preceding chapter has shown how severe calorie restriction affects the body and brain on a physiological level. This chapter deals with the way it affects the mind and thought processes.

Let's retreat for a moment and take a look at some of the reasons that motivate the need to diet. These include peer pressure, a desire to regain control over an aspect of life, or an unwanted weight gain (this applies to most people).

When you gain excess fat it usually follows a stressful incident or circumstances in your life. In the practice we have found the following to be the most common circumstances for fat gain:

- getting married
- a new baby
- domestic violence
- financial worries
- changing jobs
- loss of a loved one
- marital discord
- ongoing work pressures.

The above are all circumstances in life that cause severe stress. When these difficult situations are not dealt with correctly, by seeking counselling by a clinical therapist, confronting the problem and dealing with it, or finding support systems that can share the load, the stressor is not relieved and it is quite normal to gain weight.

The following example may sound familiar to many:

Jo is a 29-year old advertising executive. Two months ago her partner broke off the relationship and moved out. Determined not to show the world how this traumatic event has affected her life, Jo bravely carries on as if nothing has happened, dealing with the situation privately and to the best of her ability.

Many people believe that to seek help from a psychotherapist would be admitting to a weakness. As such, public stigmas associated with this type of treatment often prevent people from stopping the escalation of stress, distress and ultimate depression where they should: right from the start. Consulting with a clinical psychotherapist is immensely helpful in receiving guidance in various aspects of life, from dealing with emotions and traumatic experiences to time and stress management. A therapist provides an objective 'shoulder to cry on' while friends and relatives are usually emotionally involved. A clinical psychotherapist's role is to help you work through your feelings. Bottling up feelings will ultimately result in physical and mental illness.

Unfortunately for Jo, internalising her grief is not an effective relief for the stressor. As a result, she starts noticing a nagging feeling of disquiet and unease deep within. She ascribes this feeling to an innate weakness because no matter how hard she tries, she simply can not satisfy this strange feeling of malaise, of emptiness; this 'hole in the soul'.

The correct way to alleviate this traumatic situation would be to start professional therapy, before the stress becomes physical distress and starts affecting her. But again, this is often seen as 'the last resort, when the marbles have finally been lost', rather than a healthy choice when the effects of the stressor begin to manifest themselves in the long term. Here, Jo is feeling the beginnings of emotional distress. Her ongoing feelings of rejection are accumulating as an ongoing stress situation (remember the fight or flight response?), and she is suffering from the first signs of distress and the descent into depression. She cannot find a feeling of well-being or positiveness. She feels emotional exhaustion, because her emotional signals to deal with the situation in a healthy way are being ignored. She needs to make time to analyse the reasons for the break-up, not to blame herself entirely for the failed relationship, and try to find joy in being single and independent. However, Jo must also mourn her loss and feel the pain, instead of regarding it as a weakness to show emotion. If she fails to do this, her internalised emotions will manifest in physical symptoms. It is healthy to cry: scientists have even found stress hormones in tears, which gives a more physiological basis for the need to mourn!

Ignoring the feeling, she buries herself deeper into her work. As she increases her efforts and the hours at work, her body starts to feel the increased demands as well. Despite her efforts and supposed success, she is not rewarded with a sense of well-being as might have been expected. The 'gnawing' at her insides continues relentlessly.

Jo would rather pretend that the grief will go away and won't 'give in' to tears and mourning so that she can come to terms with the traumatic changes in her life She believes that the break-up was a result of her inadequacies. It is frightening to confront an issue that causes pain, and so she tries to fill the 'hole in her soul' (the result of not dealing with her problem). She has always been good at her work and her achievements make her feel proud. Therefore she seeks fulfilment and a much-needed boost to her confidence, working even harder to take her mind off the problem. In an attempt to fill the void with satisfaction attained from increased efforts at work, she fails to recognise that her body is already in a compromised state. It is natural for the human mind to devise intricate ways to avoid confronting an issue (as she does). However, quite the opposite happens: she will harbour these feelings within, and, like any physical need that is ignored, the urge to deal with it will become even stronger, and the negative effect on her even greater. Unfortunately for Jo, she is trying to fill a round hole with square pegs: no matter how much satisfaction she gains from her work, this cannot fill the void within, because she has not confronted, dealt with and accepted the real issues. A professional is adept at uncovering the true issues that cause the distress, and helping the patient to devise a strategy to accept the realities of the situation, to facilitate healing of the soul.

Jo has accrued some leave and decides that a holiday would probably do her good. The resort she chooses offers total seclusion and the promise of complete relaxation. Despite the lovely setting, she finds it quite difficult to unwind. Instead of enjoying the break, she spends most of her holiday anxiously thinking about all the tasks that she ostensibly left undone. She returns to work with an increased sense of pressure to work even harder and perform even better than before. Although she knows deep inside that there is, in fact, nothing that she has left undone, she still feels as though this is the case, because the 'nagging' feeling will not leave her alone, and she cannot pin-point what it is that is making her feel uneasy and guilty.

Jo begins to feel the physical signs of distress: exhaustion, inability to relax and poor self-esteem, but rationalises that they are indicative of merely too much work and not enough rest.

Unfortunately, the problem has already turned from stress to physical distress, and a short holiday will not alleviate the root cause of her problems: unresolved emotional issues. Her continued internalised mental stress would manifest itself as physical problems, regardless of the length of her holiday.

It is easier to project a problem onto something that we feel more comfortable to deal with. Confronting the break-up will cause Jo an enormous amount of pain, and so she projects the reasons for feeling the way she does onto work. If she attributes her physical feelings to overwork, there is a solution – a holiday, and a holiday is easy to deal with. Again, she's trying to fill a round hole with square pegs: the problem is not work! Low self-esteem is a very common symptom of ensuing depression, albeit deriving from a real reason, and it eventually becomes disproportionately low and pathological.

At a seminar, a wise woman partly attributed the basis of her depression to the snowball effect of all of those things left undone. She is absolutely right, in my opinion, now that we understand how stress ultimately becomes depression. The more we procrastinate over confronting an issue, the stronger the internal stressor becomes. So, the more powerful the ongoing anxiety inside, the less able we become to cope with even the smallest of stressors with which life presents us. And so the procrastinator begins to increase her anxiety about everything that she encounters, and thus her confidence in being able to cope is compromised

Her efforts at work are rewarded with a salary increase and a promotion. Yet, somehow Jo finds herself unable to let the feeling of pride and accomplishment soothe the horrible inner gnawing.

She works even harder and finds it hard to relax at night; nothing seems to help. One night she has two glasses of wine and for the first time in weeks she feels completely relaxed. Soon this becomes the only way she can wind down after a hard day's work. The drinks are her reward; something to look forward to at night.

Jo is experiencing the initial onset of depression: her body and mind are in a constant heightened fight-or-flight mode, with decreased serotonin efficacy. As a result, she feels constantly 'hyped', and begins to 'self-medicate' with alcohol. Because alcohol has very potent sedative effects, it seems logical to have a few drinks to 'calm down again'. Alcoholism is very common condition in depressive patients and is often not diagnosed as such. A depressive will not easily acknowledge 'needing' alcohol rather than 'enjoying a drink' because it signifies yet another weakness. The sedative properties of alcohol are short-lived though and the next morning the brain chemicals adapt even further. This results in even worse depressive symptoms, heightened anxiety, and ultimately results in an ongoing dependency and need to gradually increase the 'doses' of 'self-medication'. As the dependency on alcohol develops, the individual finds it difficult to admit that it has become a need. A need (or an addiction) requires 'giving up' (in this case) the one thing that successfully helped Jo to relax and feel happy again. Doing without that small piece of well-being, her life would 'feel' very difficult to cope with. So, the alcohol becomes the highlight of each day: the one special time that she feels 'normal' again – the way she felt a long time ago.

But she also develops minor ailments. The chronic headaches and niggling sinusitis are unfamiliar ailments to her. Her sleeping patterns are disturbed and she feels tired during the day. She battles to concentrate at work and finds it increasingly difficult to remember things. She seems to be the only one in the office not coping well, yet this is what she worked so hard to achieve. Nobody must know how she feels – it would be admitting failure. Ignoring what is really happening to her, she ascribes her condition to lack of sleep and increases her intake to three glasses of wine per night. Now, she is able to relax sufficiently to sleep again.

The fight-or-flight response increases continuously, partially due to unresolved issues, the mild alcohol dependency that causes physiological depression, as well as to physical and mental exhaustion. The continuous fight or flight response has caused her adrenaline to be active all the time, and this is not conducive to sleep! Depression has begun to set in biologically: the alteration in brain chemicals (largely from too little serotonin and too much adrenaline being 'felt') is causing the characteristic symptoms of lack of concentration, jumbled thought processes and poor memory.

The exhaustion prevails despite enough rest. She fears that her colleagues might notice, knowing it would spell disaster for her career. She starts taking vitamin supplements, reasoning that super-performance requires mega-doses of vitamins. The health shop becomes a regular shopping venue and slowly depletes her salary ...

Many people make this (very expensive) mistake. Some symptoms of depression are similar to those experienced from vitamin deficiencies, but regardless of the amounts of supplements taken, clinical depression cannot be cured with vitamins! In fact, often mega-doses of some vitamins can exacerbate the symptoms. For example, taking too much vitamin B complex over a long period of time has shown damage of nerve fibres. It is imperative that a professional considers all the symptoms together, to ascertain whether depression is the problem. It may not be a deficiency disease at all! Because the symptoms are numerous, the sufferer will often choose not to reveal them all to a doctor for fear and shame of sounding like a hypochondriac.

Having enough rest will not alleviate depressive exhaustion, because there is a pathological imbalance of brain chemicals, not a lack of sleep! Remember that her brain is registering incorrect signals from this imbalance, making her 'feel' as though she needs to fight or flee all the time. This is exhausting to the mind, as well as damaging to the body. Such persistent heightened anxiety (even if it has no immediate cause, as in this situation) wreaks havoc on all of the body organs, including her immunity. As a result, her body's immune system suffers: it becomes susceptible to colds, flu and other minor infections, as well as becoming allergic to other substances such as pollen, animal hair, etc. Such allergies are often unfamiliar to the sufferer, further illustrating that the body's functions are no longer normal.

To fight the exhaustion and stay awake, Jo increases her caffeine intake from the usual one or two cups, to eight cups of coffee per day. Because of her workload she eats on the run most days. Lately she craves sweet things and reasons that a few chocolates are quite harmless, seeing that she eats so little anyway.

A vicious circle

Jo is unaware of the vicious circle that threatens to destroy her sanity and health:

As a result of permanent exhaustion, she 'self-medicates' with an 'upper', namely caffeine. Caffeine accentuates the activity of adrenaline, which makes her feel more alert and temporarily conquers the tiredness caused by the depression. However, by increasing the activity of the very substance that she already is so sensitive to (adrenaline), it is evident that the depression will intensify over time. She feels the 'kick' of caffeine, but this is followed by a decrease in blood sugar levels, causing a 'slump'. Consequently she needs another cup of coffee and the process of 'up' and 'down' is repeated. Soon she will develop a caffeine dependency, characterised by persistent headaches unless she has more coffee. Painkillers alleviate the headaches, but they usually have a sedative effect that further stimulates the need for caffeine to 'keep going'. This will often result in a dependency on pain-killers as well. This type of addiction is very common, but if the underlying problems are to be treated successfully, they have to be diagnosed correctly.

Secondly, because the caffeine increases her body's sensitivity to adrenaline, her serotonin dysfunction becomes even more appar-ent, and the anxiety and depression intensify. Moreover, her sugar levels are on a roller coaster ride, increasing the serotonin dysfunc-tion. To overcome this problem, she intuitively 'self-medicates' with carbohydrates, choosing high-calorie fatty foods (her body believes that it is in a famine situation again, because of her plummeting sugar levels), and high GI carbohydrates. These will flood her blood with sugar, thus indirectly stimulating increased serotonin produc-tion to make her feel better.

Jo assumes that her body will burn the calories from the choco-lates and crisps like before. But she is wrong! She notices a gradual increase in her body fat despite eating only a little. Lately, she has had to buy her clothes one size larger, and she also retains a lot of water.

Remember that when the body is in a state of persistent anxi-ety, or depression, the ongoing cortisol production can cause insulin resistance. This means that the blood sugar levels are of-ten high, but so are the insulin levels (trying to store all the blood sugar). However, the insulin cannot function properly. Remem-ber that insulin stores! As fat from fatty foods is absorbed into the bloodstream, it will immediately be stored! Her metabolism no longer reacts like before, even though she eats fewer calories in total. Due to the chemical changes in her body, she is now in perpetual storage mode. Consequently, her body stores almost any fat that she eats! Moreover, because there is so much insulin in her blood, indirectly she will also 'store' water, hence the increased water retention.

Her menstrual cycle becomes irregular (a result of the immense hormonal changes that occur with the HPA axis being 'out of kilter') and she often has a sore throat. She also develops eczema and other nagging allergies, such as rhinitis, a bloated stomach and itchy eyes, and feels uglier and more useless than before.

Despite the supplements, Jo feels out of control. Her body is not coping with the stress, her performance at work leaves much to be desired, and she has lost interest in all the things she enjoyed before. Her self-confidence has retreated behind a wall of insecurity and she feels so emotionally 'raw' that the smallest jibe causes an emotional outburst – either irrational anger or tears. She reacts with venomous aggression to kindness and care, and distances herself from anyone who threatens to expose her vulnerability. Caring little for anyone else's needs, she devotes all her time and energy to keep going.

This, in turn, decreases her stress level, which in turn reduces her ability to function smoothly. So, she avoids and procrastinates more and more, and she finds she cannot finish any job, of those she has managed to tackle. So, her feelings of inadequacy and guilt are so enormous, that this adds to the stress levels, and drives the nail deeper. What's more, her awareness of how much she is disappointing everybody increases, and makes her raw with guilt. Somebody tells her that she must just pull herself together, and stop being so stupid – but no one knows this more acutely than she does! She agrees, and starts a habit of apologising for everything that she does, in the hope that she can prove to all around her that she knows she is useless, and that she is not oblivious to her incompetence to merely be a deserving human being.

Can you see how she starts the power-struggle of apologies; trying to get in there first to prove to everyone that she knows she is worthless, before they have time to tell her themselves. And from being a control freak one moment, she becomes a clinging, needy and child-like creature, apathetic to her own sense of dignity, and desperate to grasp at any attention or care she can get. Her ultimate obsession is to curl up into a ball, and shut the world out. All shreds of confidence in being able to get up and start again have disintegrated. She doesn't even want to any more. Every time she does anything, it is foolish, embarrassing, out of control, childish, stupid and ugly. She feels like a burden to herself, let alone anyone else, and her will to continue has vanished.

She has reached rock bottom. Her body has finally shown her that it will win over her mind.

Her increasing weight causes her to feel emotionally depressed, but the underlying clinical depression leads to hallmark symptoms of a chemical imbalance: aggression, ongoing feelings of guilt (albeit devoid of reason), social withdrawal, and lack of energy and interest in previously pleasurable activities.

Horrified, Jo guiltily puts her inexplicable behaviour down to incompetence and failure at work. In an effort to meet the impossible goals she has set for herself, she drinks more coffee and eats less during the day, drinks more wine at night to relax and sleep, and works even harder. Without consideration for her ability to meet these goals, she soldiers on. Jo knows that she has no choice. If she fails now she will lose everything that she holds most dear, as well as her sense of self-worth; failing will only confirm her greatest fear – that she is not good enough. She feels she wasn't good enough for her relationship, and now the one thing she has always felt confident in (work) is also becoming a symbol of her failure.

At this point, matters take a turn for the worse. Jo's soul desperately cries for warm creature comforts and demands to be isolated from everything associated with responsibility. She succumbs to her innermost call for nourishment. However, instead of feeding her soul with emotional therapy, she eats. Once started, it is impossible to stop and she comforts herself with chocolate cake, bread glistening with butter and peanut butter, ice cream ... The food makes her feel like a child again as she remembers a time when others took care of her and comforted her.

The carbohydrates Jo eats stimulate the serotonin production her body has been without for so long, but they also stimulate the powerful storage hormone, insulin. Her comfort foods are not made up of carbohydrates alone, though, and the insulin stores carbohydrates and fats. Great amounts of fat are carried silently into her bloodstream, and the insulin directs it promptly to her thighs or buttocks.

She enters a new cycle: one of binge-guilt and starvation. This only serves to reinforce her feelings of being out of control, as well as giving her more ammunition with which to hate her already out-of-control body. Each time she puts anything into her mouth, she cannot control herself, and this only makes her fat. Each time she drinks, she makes a fool of herself or gets into trouble. And each time she tries anything, her deep-seated sense of inadequacy results in her doing things in a half-hearted manner.

WHEN YOU FEEL INADEQUATE, YOUR PERFORMANCE WILL NEVER BE BETTER THAN JUST ADEQUATE. THE HUMAN MIND HAS THE POWER TO SET EMOTIONAL LIMITS TO ONE'S CAPABILITIES. BECAUSE JO IS FEELING INADEQUATE, SHE WILL NOT BELIEVE THAT SHE CAN DO WELL, AND SO THEREFORE SHE WON'T.

She feels as though she has completely lost control over her body. She consults others to help her decide on matters concerning her life, fearing that she is inadequate to make correct decisions. Her feelings of inadequacy prevent her from making any of her own decisions eventually, and when she allows others to decide on important matters on her behalf, these feelings are further reinforced.

She cannot drink in moderation, because she 'needs' to relax. Alcohol seems to be the only thing that makes her relax. She fights with feelings of 'deserving' the relaxation, but while she is trying to relax (sleeping, drug or alcohol abuse), all she can do is reinforce how she cannot live without these things – that she is useless.

She cannot control her eating, and her needs and eating habits no longer resemble those of a 'normal' person. So she feels even more alienated and worthless. Her attempts at 'controlling' her eating choices and amounts simply crash with the first temptation of food, and so her 'control' aspirations are again weakened.

So, she seeks the help of a 'diet' from a slimming club.

When seeking help for a weight problem, it is necessary to seek the help of a professional trained in such a field, i.e. a registered, clinical dietician. Slimming clubs have helped many people to lose weight, but unfortunately, they do not usually have the trained professionals able to differentiate whether or not an obesity problem is due to food or another, more deep-seated problem, such as hormonal imbalances and depression (almost impossible to detect with any blood tests). People are attracted to a diet club rather than a dietician because of the all-too-frequent apparent success of a friend who loses quickly on the relevant programme. Losing fat (not muscle) safely and successfully in the long term means being patient and allowing the body to heal what may be wrong, as well as maintaining health. This takes time, and because of the desperate need to lose weight immediately to alleviate the poor self-esteem associated with being over-fat, people are drawn to quick fixes. They are often successful in the short term, but now that we understand what harm they can do to the body and brain, it is time that we take fat loss seriously. Simply following a calorie-controlled eating plan that differs very little from person to person usually results in a problem such as Jo is experiencing becoming much more serious.

In my opinion, slimming clubs that advocate restrictive eating simply reinforce the dysfunctional mind patterns of not being able to 'control oneself', and needing to be 'told' how much one is allowed. This reinforces feelings of being completely out of control.

Moreover, Jo will not lose weight successfully while she suffers from clinical depression, because one of the effects of cortisol is to cause insulin resistance. By eating fewer calories, she will become even more insulin resistant, and her serotonin production will decrease further. This entire process increases the organic basis for clinical depression and apart from destroying any self-confidence she may have left; she will also develop increasingly powerful cravings for fatty and starchy foods to 'self-medicate' her depression. Diet clubs often fail to teach dieters about the fat content of various foods. When they consume hidden fats (which are inevitably stored) in fits of desperation, the result is usually a scolding at the next weigh-in.

The mounting shame associated with these 'cheats' lowers the self-esteem even further. Club leaders may also perceive the cheat as much bigger than the dieter confesses to.

I have so often witnessed the tears and desperate pleadings of many obese patients to be believed that despite eating moderately, they still get fat. I share their pain (as if obesity isn't enough of a social stigma to contend with without having to be called a liar), and bitter anger at how they are treated by 'experts' who still believe that obesity is caused simply by overeating.

Obesity does not have a single cause: it is one of the most challenging epidemics in the world today. More people die from obesity than heart attacks and cancer combined.

My personal experience leads me to believe that depression accounts for the majority of metabolic abnormalities associated with weight gain. And I mean the physiological changes in the body's handling of food, not only the obvious and 'shameful' comfort eating.

Treating obesity by starving, in my opinion, is the worst thing to do. Being overweight is the body's way of conveying a message that there is an innate imbalance. It is not healthy being overweight, but starvation for the sake of losing that weight is doubly harmful:

- Firstly, it mounts the stressors in the body: that of hunger as well as other stressors (hunger is an extremely powerful stressor).
- Secondly, it is like an override button: regardless of any underlying problems, the only aim is to get thin. This will result in a temporary thinness only, because for every day that the hunger signals are ignored, the rebound action of mounting stressors becomes increasingly powerful.

Those who fear lack of control, such as people with tendencies towards anorexia or bulimia nervosa, will surely be enticed into this controlled environment. When they are given these parameters, their fear of failure and lack of self-trust urges them to simply stay well within those boundaries – to move slightly faster than everyone else not as a race, but as a means of ensuring that they have a safety net for when they ultimately fail.

When their diet plan suggests a cup of rice, for instance, they will insist on having just less than a cup, because they feel that they can't trust themselves anyway! The resultant 'successes' (by getting thinner and thinner, and finding increasing ways to improve the system) they experience only serve to fuel the fire of self-destruction, because by that stage the small sense of success serves to partially fill the void, and they want more.

But they never reach that point of inner satisfaction and peace. This can only be attained once they are confident that they have enough self-control to eat moderately.

Jo's descent into this spiral of events was caused by not mourning her failed relationship and by concealing her grief and anger. By joining a diet club her pathology will be made worse, to the point where she is no longer in a position to logically understand what needs to be done.

Her mounted stress response is so powerful, now, that she devotes her entire body's energy into taking every conceivable measure she can to not give in to her body's own signals. She is hungry – no, starving, and yet she cannot eat, now: she has gained weight, and so she must eat less! If she eats more than what is 'allowed' she will fail and get fat again. In fact, if she ever listens to her body again, she will gain weight, so she must do anything and everything to ignore her hunger pangs and anxiety.

At some time or other, her body stops giving. She either reaches breaking point as the descent into chronic illness affects her whole life, gradually losing friends, loved ones, and even a sense of herself, whilst withdrawing from all responsibility for her own actions (like getting drunk regularly), or she has a nervous breakdown. Either way, the damage done to her loved ones as well as to herself can be crippling. It may even catalyse thoughts about and attempts to commit suicide.

Jo has turned to friends and family to help her overcome this destructive pattern and in turn they step in to 'save' her. This develops into a spiral of co-dependency: Jo feels that their support is imperative to her existence and success, and they believe that their own sense of self-worth is inadequate unless they can save her from this turmoil.

The co-dependency becomes pathological, often leading to the end of a relationship or an unexpected and sudden jolt into reality. Remember, we humans aren't good compromisers and moderators, are we?

Jo has succumbed to the controlling environment of the dieting mentality. She no longer trusts her own body. She believes that she is a failure unless she eats according to what is 'prescribed' by someone who must know her body better than she does. She begins to fear food in all of its aspects. She fears being hungry, and sees this natural physical signal as being something 'wrong' and that which must be fought against. She moves away from understanding and respecting her body. She fears that which is tasty, or even that which brings pleasure. She associates food with guilt, and pleasure with weakness. She has dieted herself into depression (both emotionally and organically, by altering her brain chemicals and the functioning of her body), and truly believes that she deserves to feel this bad.

The dieting mentality shows itself in many ways. Read the following comments made by people with a typical dieting mentality and find out if your thinking patterns have also been altered by calorie cutting:

'I can't have any gravies, they're fattening!' Despite the fact that we tell you they can be fat free!

'Sugar! Never! It is so loaded with calories!' Even though sugar cannot make you fat.

'I am so good: I hardly ever eat starches and carbohydrates!' Your poor body has no fuel!

'I can't tell you what I ate yesterday! It's so bad!' Even though it actually isn't that bad.

'I love salad with nothing on it besides vinegar!' When you are really hungry, a tart salad is not the most satisfying meal if you are honest with yourself. Besides, never in my years of being a dietician, have I ever heard anybody saying that they were so hungry, that they ate a whole salad to themselves!

'A plain baked potato with nothing on it is fine.' No it isn't! Your tastebuds want interesting flavours and your mouth likes to feel different textures. Pretending that something this plain is acceptable means that you have not accepted that eating healthily must last for a lifetime. Plain baked potatoes won't keep you happy for the rest of your life. Eventually you will turn to something that has real flavour and texture, such as a packet of crisps, or a large steak with cheese sauce.

'I know I have tomato pasta every night, but I love it.' You may love it now, but it shows me that you are still too frightened to try anything that may "look" fatty, even if it isn't. Again, having tomato pasta for the next 30 years will turn even Pavarotti against pasta for good!

'I like plain food.' Why then, do you go to restaurants?

'I don't feel nice when I'm full.' You should! Physiologically, we are meant to eat until we are full. Mentally, you have been well trained into thinking that you don't need to feel that. Yes you do!

'But bananas are so fattening! They are so sweet!' They are not fattening, and sweetness has nothing to do with gaining fat.

Many people have learnt to love salads and fruits as a staple, by denying their honest needs for warm, tasty foods. Others have gone to the other extreme: they hate fruits and vegetables because they associate them with the only things they are 'allowed'. Again, these are a healthy part of a diet, which should be eaten every day, in addition to other foods. Too much of a good thing stops it being good.

Because the dieting mentality seems to afflict more women than men, I usually ask my female patients to listen to the wants of their male friends and family members. Words like, 'I want real meals, not this rabbit food!' brings a huge sigh of relief to me. Thank heavens some people are honest about what their bodies really want! And we ought to give it to ourselves – in a way that leaves no room for comment (even if it is fat free, you should be the only one who needs to know it). Food should not taste 'healthy', it should taste good. If you eat only 'healthy-tasting' food you will either eventually succumb to the 'naughty' foods, or adapt your mental attitude so vigorously into accepting that you actually enjoy bland food. This is what I call dysfunctional because it is ignoring a very natural need to enjoy things.

Weight gain is still seen as gluttony, and this induces ongoing feelings of guilt. Strict diets seem to be the only 'way out' and yet it has been proven that they do not work because they ignore most of the reasons for weight gain. Furthermore, they induce mental and physiological needs that are seen as 'bad' or 'naughty'. The metabolism is also changed (metabolic muscle-mass decreases as well as insulin resistance promoting fat storage), and so rebound fat-gain becomes inevitable and natural, as the body struggles to survive. This reinforces the depression felt by the diet-induced depressive, and causes a life-long obsession and fear of food, as well as decreasing health, as the body appears to spiral out of control. Actually, if we look past the dieting mentality, and peer deep into the natural workings of the body, becoming preoccupied with food is clearly the most perfect and natural survival technique to prevent us from dying of starvation.

No longer may we view the obese body as one that is weak and gluttonous. We must now see it exactly as it is: one that is struggling to survive. It has employed a millennia-old technique to protect itself against starvation. It has prepared itself beautifully to cope with anxiety, fight and flight, and ongoing trauma. The more we harm it (starvation is harmful to the body – it is an unpleasant and traumatic physical affliction), the more it ensures that we will be OK – it stores energy for such circumstances. The more harmful the circumstances it encounters, the more it will adapt to protect us in the best way it knows how. And we shun these survival techniques as being naughty!

Here ends the dieting mentality for good.

Here begins giving the body what it deserves: good food, happy meals, celebration of its survival, and most of all: appreciation for what it has done for us in response for how little we have done for it.

I want you to make a promise to your body out loud, and with the triumph you and your body deserve as a team that has survived through thick and thin:

'I will never put you through a famine again. I will never put you through such trauma again. I will now listen to you, and give you what you need: love, cherishing and respect. I will show you that we will never again endure starvation, bland food or self-admonishment. We will now enter a new life of enjoyment together, and I will work to find the untreated problems, and treat them. I will heal you and will love being inside you from now on. Forever. Thank you, body, for seeing me through all of these hard times.

'I am sorry for having put you through them.'

12 DIETETIC TREATMENT

So, now you understand that dieting is, quite simply, bad for you – and worsens the problem of a high body fat content. You also know that depression is very common, and fairly easily treated, when you know how. By now you will also realise that restrictive dieting can indirectly lead to depression, and that depression more often than not leads to fat gain. You are now fully equipped to put your knowledge to good use, but this is often easier said than done. And this is where I, as a dietician, can help.

I will now move through each of The X Clinic's food groups, which differ from the standard food groups because they relate differently, according to their metabolic effects. I will then move on to eating patterns and attitudes, and then how these relate to such behaviours as craving and bingeing.

Carbohydrates

One of the most important parts of dietetic therapy with regard to weight control and psychiatric illness is blood sugar control. Remember that when I speak of sugar, it includes all carbohydrates. We need carbohydrates because they are all made of glucose (a type of sugar), which our bodies need a constant supply of, in order to remain alive. So, we eat carbohydrates, and they 'dissolve' into sugar into our bloodstreams. This is our 'petrol', and keeps us going. When there are changes in the concentration of this sugar in the blood, there are direct effects on the rest of the body, including the brain. The sugar concentration in the blood depends on many things, including times of eating, how much is eaten, and what type of carbohydrates are eaten. This re-introduces the subject of the Glycaemic Index of carbohydrates, or the GI.

High GI carbohydrates dissolve into sugar very quickly, thus increasing the blood sugar level rapidly, with a large amount of energy present for utilisation. This typically lasts only a short time, because insulin is released to 'store' it into the muscles where it can be used for energy. However, in people who are insulin resistant, this insulin cannot exert its effects capably, because the insulin 'doors' into the muscle won't open to insulin. Thus, in order for the blood sugar level to decrease again as it should (the energy needs to be in the muscles, not waiting in the blood), the body has to produce more insulin than normal. Thus, the blood sugar levels behave normally, in terms of filling with sugar, and then emptying again, but much more insulin is needed to effect this.

Remember that insulin means storing, and this is in direct opposition to burning/losing, so fat loss (despite dieting) becomes difficult in insulin resistance. This is why eating high GI carbohydrates won't make you fat, but they won't make you thin either. They will just keep you the same, which is often not the desired effect in someone who is overweight from depression! Remember that it is the excessive cortisol released in depression that effects this insulin resistance. It is also the reason why people who have never had a weight problem before, start gaining weight during and after periods of depression. It makes you insulin resistant, which turns you, quite literally, into a storage machine! So: avoid high GI foods until the depression has been dealt with professionally, or unless you are of healthy size and do not need to lose body fat.

The best way to go is to stick with as low GI carbohydrates as you can. These are the carbohydrates which dissolve more slowly into sugar into the blood so that they have much less need for insulin, and therefore lessen the 'storage' message being delivered to the insulin-resistant body.

Of course, the Glycaemic Index is only a guide to help us understand the relative speed with which carbohydrates deliver sugar to the blood, and is not meant to be a list of hard-and-fast numbers to which everyone reacts identically. Some people will experience greater or smaller sugar changes with the same GI carbohydrates as other people, and so exact numbers are often difficult to determine for an entire population. But, the numbers serve as a guide, to allow us to understand which ones are better at slowing down sugar release than others, and to use the GI as a powerful tool for sugar control.

GLYCAEMIC INDEX EXCHANGE

Carbohydrate	GI
Cornflakes/ Rice Crispies/ Mealie meal	100
White/ Brown/ Wholewheat/ French bread	100
Honey	100
Puffed Wheat	100
Weet Bix	100
Potato – mashed	100
Potato – baked	100
Crispbread	89
Rye bread	89
Instant rice	87
Rice cakes	81
Potato – boiled	80
Coco Pops/ Frosties	77
Bagel	72
Gnocchi	68
Oatso Easy	66
Brown rice	66
Peas, green	65
Cous cous	61
Sweet corn (plain or creamed)	60
Baked beans	60
Ryvita/ Finn Crisp	59
Cane sugar	59
Basmati rice	58
Haricot beans	57
All Bran flakes/ Special K	54
White rice – parboiled	54
Oats porridge	47
Potato, Sweet	46
Butter beans	46
Chick peas	40
Pasta (all types, cooked al dente)	40
Lentils	28
Fructose	22
Pearled barley	22
Soy beans/ soy mince	21

Taken from *The GI Factor,* by Dr J Brand Miller.

The most important thing to remember when GI manipulating ('GIMming'), is that the food must be delicious. It is so common for people to get stuck in the dieting mentality and feel 'pious' when eating boiled lentils and pearled barley. This is not food! This is medicine, and food should be fun! After years of knowing that eating bland food is associated with weight loss, people still think that the more tasteless the food is, the quicker they will lose weight. WRONG! The food must be fantastic, and delicious, to ensure that you want to eat like this for a very long time to come, indeed. So, haul out **The X Diet Cookbook**, and start making bobotie and lasagne, chicken à la king and creamy curries, and enjoy low GI foods the way they are supposed to be enjoyed!

Not only do low GI carbohydrates minimise the insulin-induced 'storage' message, thereby allowing more efficient fat loss, but they also keep the blood sugar level constant, rather than putting us on a sugar roller-coaster. Remember that when the sugar levels are constant, so is the brain's production of serotonin, thus reducing significantly the bouts of anxiety and depression experienced when sugar levels drop. Remember that when our sugar levels dip, we experience feelings of depression – which are worsened if you have clinical depression or are simply pre-menstrual. Remember that when the sugar levels are low in the blood (after not eating enough, having not eaten for too long a period of time, or having eaten a high GI carbohydrate which didn't last long enough to sustain you), the entry of tryptophan into the brain is reduced. This, in turn, reduces the amount of serotonin produced, thereby reducing the 'controlling' effect serotonin has on the brain and body. So, the aim is to try and keep the sugar levels as constant as possible, without letting them drop.

High GI carbohydrates would induce rise-and-drop phases, with chances of sugar levels dropping after eating them, so despite the fact that they tend to make us feel better, we end up feeling worse almost immediately afterwards. Low GI carbohydrates, however, keep the blood sugar level low, reducing insulin production and ensuring a constant and steady supply of sugar to the blood to prevent dips. Thus, the clinically depressed person will not be 'cured' of their depression by eating low GI foods, but it certainly prevents 'bad' times experienced after sugar dips.

Remember, too, that in clinical depression, there are very often gastro-intestinal problems such as spastic colon and constipation. Eating enough carbohydrates will help regulate this, due to their content of soluble and insoluble fibres. Both have differing effects on the colon, but both are equally important, and by maintaining adequate 'bulk' of food quantity in the colon, more regular stools will automatically be induced.

Fats

Please understand one very important issue, here. Fats are not bad! In fact, all foods have their place, with respect to whatever therapeutic dietary prescription is being dealt with. Chocolates are not bad! They are unsuitable for someone trying to lose fat, but very important for an athlete. Brown bread is very good for someone with mild constipation, but not at all good for someone trying to lose fat (it is high GI), and with a spastic colon (it is full of insoluble fibre). A baked potato is wonderful for someone who has no disorders, but terrible for someone with diabetes.

You see, all food is good, but I concentrate on fat loss and Syndrome X, in which arena the patient's body is terrible at coping with fats! So, although all fats play their part in a normal, healthy lifestyle where no therapeutic effects of nutrition are needed to treat a disorder, fats as a whole are completely unsuitable in an insulin-resistant body whose main symptom is to store every bit of fat it comes into contact with! So, remove the fats entirely, for therapeutic treatment of the disorder, get the body right, and then get back to eating fats again, once the body is better!

Insulin resistance can be minimised and even controlled to the point of absence, but it does warrant special and ongoing monitoring if fats are to be included – especially if it is tied up with the concurrent disorder of depression, with its insulin-resistant cortisol production. Medication, psychotherapy and a reasonable alteration in lifestyle will keep depression at bay such that you are completely 'better', but enter another life stressor (which is just life!) and the depression may rear its head again, and cause insulin resistance to worsen, thereby necessitating removal of fats again. It really is as simple as that. While the body is unwell for some reason, treat it carefully by preventing it storing fats! Then, when the problem is under control, go back to a low-fat but not necessarily fat-free diet.

So, you see, fats are not bad, and you will never hear a dietician saying that any foodstuff is bad for you: all foods just have different functions in the body, and when those functions are disrupted, we simply remove the fats to prevent them from interfering with that disruption. When we remove a whole food group like this, however, we need to give the body back the vital nutrients which may be lost in the process: in this case, the vital nutrients found in some fats are essential fatty acids. These can be supplemented using the concentrated essential fats in the form of a supplement, such as evening primrose oil and salmon oil capsules. Thus, we still get the essential components into the body, without the 'extra' fats they would normally be found in, which would otherwise be stored in insulin resistance.

So, getting down to insulin resistance, supplements should be taken, and intake of fats should be eliminated as best possible. This can be very difficult, because fats are actually hidden in most foods. Therefore, we at The X Clinic have stipulated an easy-to-follow rule of eating foods with less than 3 g of fat per 100 g serving. Clearly, there will still be fats included in the diet, so strictly speaking we cannot call it fat free – a modicum of liberty is involved. So, whenever we call anything fat free, please bear in mind that it is not literally fat free, but very nearly so!

Following a fat-free diet such as this means not just cutting out butter, margarine and fried foods! In fact, in the bigger scope of things, this would only be effective in reducing the fat intake by about half – which is still good, but not good enough for a disorder such as insulin resistance. We have to learn to be 'fat sleuths', looking at everything we eat, not for the calorie content as we used to, because that is now irrelevant, but for the fat content of all foods. Harmless, 'healthy' foods contain many nutrients, one of them often being fats! For instance, a bran muffin contains up to 25% fats! So, trusting our instincts on fats is not always effective: we need to look and see for ourselves!

Remember that the value for foods should always be per 100 g serving. Otherwise, we may trustingly accept that a food satisfies the less than 3 g of fat part, only to find that it is actually per 10 g serving, rendering it a sly 30 g/100 g! In the same light, don't automatically walk past 'fattening'-looking foodstuffs such as drinking chocolate: one brand actually contains less than 2 g of fat per 100 g serving!

Cooking fat free is not easy, either. In fact, many people try and be terribly pious by boiling, steaming or dry-grilling foods, which may render them fat free, but oh boy! – it can be tasteless! Even frying onions in a little oil is forbidden for someone with insulin resistance, but trying to simmer onions in water is completely awful as a base to a meal! This is why I have devised ***The X Diet Cookbook***, which teaches you to dry-fry onions, using stock water and wine (or apple juice if wine is unsuitable for other reasons), allowing us to still enjoy dark brown, caramelised onions just as if we were using fat, but with no trace of it at all!

Most of the recipes I have devised have not only been attempted about seven times to ensure that they taste just like the real thing, but also have been tested on the most discerning of eaters: middle-aged men! Please be careful about trying to cook fat-free on your own; following your own instincts and hoping they will turn out as good as the real thing will usually barely suffice. But food is not meant to be merely sufficient! It is meant to be anticipated and celebrated! So, please don't settle for good enough for a diet, ensure that every meal is one that is good enough for the rest of your friends and family; then it will be good enough for you to follow for a long time. Remember, you do not 'go on diet', you change your lifestyle to a healthy one, which is enjoyable, easy and long-term.

So, start your 'fat sleuthing': ask your dietician, doctor or pharmacist for the correct amount of essential fatty acids for your body, and away you go!

Proteins

These are the building blocks of the body, and are needed for many functions, the chief of which is muscle maintenance. However, most people eat too much protein when trying to maintain or build muscle. The amount of animal protein needed to fuel adequate muscle building is actually equivalent to about 1-2 chicken breast fillets per day! This is because proteins don't only come from animal meats, they also come from most other foods you eat, such as most carbohydrates, dairies and so on.

Westerners usually rely on an animal protein for each main meal, simply because it is a cultural choice. It is important not to change such cultural choices too much, so this is why the very low-fat animal proteins are acceptable, such as chicken breast fillets (the other parts of chicken are too fatty), and white fish (hake, haddock, tuna in water and kabeljou, among others). Red meat is generally too fatty, even if you can't see the fat. So, we recommend venison and ostrich (without visible fat). This type of red meat is still enjoyable, and yet does not contain as much hidden fat as ordinary beef or lamb. Pork and veal are also not too bad in their fat content, but we still recommend staying away from them.

Remember, as mentioned above, not to cook proteins in a boring way: they should continue to be an important part of your diet if they have been before. So, cut the chicken into strips and dry-fry with the onions, then add fat free sauces and gravies (see **The X Diet Cookbook**). Try, also, to stick to your old recipe favourites, such as 'stroganoff' and 'à la king', but just make them fat free. Again, see the **Cookbook** for correct ways to keep the flavour as good!

An interesting new discovery with respect to nutrition and depression, is that proteins rich in the amino acid tryptophan may help reduce symptoms of depression. It is proposed that this would occur by increasing the amount of available tryptophan in the blood, to form serotonin (tryptophan is the precursor to serotonin). Unfortunately, this is still in the embryonic stages of research, because it is very difficult to obtain proteins which have enough tryptophan in them to override the competition it experiences in the blood to become serotonin (see previous chapters for more detail). So, for the moment, simply eating a normal amount of proteins with the correct amounts of low GI carbohydrates will ensure the same result, with no added complications!

Also, as mentioned before, high protein/low carbohydrate diets are actually detrimental to the disorder of depression, because they alter the brain chemicals dramatically. So, again, a diet that appears to work immediately may be working against the very problem often causing the overweight state – that is, depression – so that when you have reached your 'goal', you are in a worse mental state than when you began, and you are much more prone to gaining more fat thereafter. So, keeping a level head about it is always the best bet, unless, of course, the damage has been done, and your head is 'not so level' any more! Get to eating happily again, won't you?!

Polish foods

These are the group that delivers all the vitamins and minerals our bodies need for correct all-over functioning. This is why we should eat many of them. In fact, most people don't eat enough for truly good health, so increasing these amounts is always a welcome instruction. Check for yourself if you eat plenty of the following polish foods:

- fruits (fresh and dried)
- vegetables (fresh and frozen)
- salads
- fat-free dairy (remember, these must be fat free: the 3 g/100 g-rule does not apply to dairies, they must simply be labelled 'fat free').

None of these contains fats (except avocado and nuts and seeds, which should be avoided), and so they can be eaten freely and happily by those following an insulin-resistant diet. They contain some sugars and are thus classified as carbohydrates, but in this instance you are free to ignore this knowledge completely, because the amount of carbohydrate they contain is relatively negligible. For instance, a food must yield 15 g of carbohydrate in order to be called a carbohydrate. For instance, 1 slice of bread yields about 15 g of carbohydrate, and so this is one serving of carbohydrate. Bananas, for instance, would have to be eaten by the bunch in order to yield 15 g of carbohydrate! We can safely say that fruits do not count as a carbohydrate in this instance, so keep them classified as a polish food, because that is what all of these foods do to the body: they polish everything up, keeping it all in good, shiny working order! So, if you feel the need to eat four oranges at once, enjoy! The vitamins and minerals being delivered to your body are invaluable!

However, please remember that these foods are not sufficient as a meal. Just as you not only fill up your car with petrol, but also get oil, water and anti-freeze, so you should get your carbohydrate-petrol, and 'polish' up your body with the oil and water equivalents: the polish foods! Always remember that good old word: balance! Always include as many polish foods with each meal as you can, and you will automatically get enough vitamins, minerals and fibre to keep that petrol being burned effectively!

Eating patterns and attitudes

I wish eating were a simple and enjoyable part of one's life, and not filled with complications – but the dieting revolution has altered our perceptions of food and eating. This must stop! Few people can start a diet without making mistakes or exceptions to the rule. This is normal behaviour, and is nothing to worry about. Unfortunately, though, slimming clubs have effectively made people feel guilty for having 'cheated', as if making a mistake is a sin!

Food should never, ever, make you feel guilty. There is generally a profound reason for deviation from the 'perfect' regimen. People crave foods, and the feeling is usually so overwhelming that they act upon it. Then, because they know that it is not what was 'supposed' to have happened, they feel like a naughty child! This is not the case! The body is so magnificent that it tells us what is happening inside of it. Most of the time it self-medicates correctly. For instance, if you are in the hot sun, and are becoming dehydrated, your body will automatically tell you what needs to happen: you will move to the shade, you will go and get a glass of water, and will want to lie down to get your blood pressure back to normal again.

The same thing happens with food: if your sugar levels drop for whatever reason, you will feel hungry. This must be obeyed! Then, if sugar levels are changing because of another reason – you have depression, for instance – your body will automatically have a strong physiological need for something that will help increase the inadequate serotonin levels in the brain. The foods it will need are high GI carbohydrates, which indirectly increase serotonin production, thereby making you feel better!

Unfortunately, unqualified 'gurus' tell you to avoid these foods, because they believe, incorrectly, that they will cause you to put on weight. So, the body is forced to ignore its signals, thereby opening itself up to the physiological abnormality. I mean, if you were very hot and thirsty in the sun, and someone told you to not drink, and to stay there, you would at least have the sense to know that you should listen first to your body's signals! So why don't you listen to your body's signals with food needs?

One of the most important things I can tell my patients is to relax! – enjoy food, and listen to the body. If your body's signals are intense and persistent, then keep listening, but understand that they may be ongoing signals of a deeper meaning, about a more deep-seated physical problem. For instance, if you keep being thirsty, no matter how much you drink, then you may have diabetes, or a kidney problem. So, don't stop drinking water, deal with the problem! In the same light, if your body keeps needing sweet things, then don't deprive yourself of sweet things, because your body needs them. But, while you are eating the sweet things, consult someone about why this keeps happening, and you may find that it is a symptom of clinical depression.

The old attitudes to food that must change are:

- 'Ignore hunger signals; you don't really need the food!'
- 'Sweet things are fattening.'
- 'A need for sweet things is a "sugar addiction".' There is no such thing, because you cannot be addicted to something the human body needs.
- 'You must always measure out the amounts of food you should eat, because if you listen to your body, you will get fat.'
- 'The less you eat, the thinner you will get.'
- 'The less you eat, the better.'
- 'Eating fibrous things makes you feel full, so that you won't want to eat for a while afterwards.' (Why try and kid your body? It needs what it is asking for!)
- 'Eating less will make your stomach "shrink", which will make eating less easy.' (Again, why try and trick your body into eating less than it needs?)

- 'Eating a big meal is bad for you.' (If your body wants a big meal sometimes, then it needs it! If you are never satisfied, however, find out if there is an underlying problem such as a psychological food obsession, for instance. If this is the case, continue giving your body what it needs until such time as the psychological aspect has been dealt with, and then you will settle down to a normal eating pattern without even trying.)
- 'People get fat because they eat too much.' (Remember amounts are rarely the problem: an underlying disorder is, and so is the types of foods interacting with their particular metabolic condition.)
- 'A good appetite is something to be ashamed of and controlled.'
- 'Deprivation is what fat people deserve.'

These should be replaced with:

- I love food!
- I love feeling satisfied at the end of a good meal.
- Food is very important to me.
- Food plays an integral part of my day-to-day life; I love preparing good food, and I love sharing it with friends and family.
- I am proud of having a good appetite.
- I enjoy a good indulgence every now and then – it helps make occasions that much more special.
- I trust my body's signals, and I will co-operate with it when these signals indicate something other than daily changes in appetite.
- My body needs different things at different times, and so long as my diet always has a good balance of carbohydrates, polish foods and proteins, I will satisfy those needs.
- I will not settle for anything less than delicious food at all times.
- I understand that being overfat is a symptom of a body that is not well, and that it should be cared for, not punished.
- When I get bad influenza, I make life easier for myself by going to bed and accepting care from others until I am better. When I am overweight, I will afford myself the same care, and make my life easier (for instance by enjoying good and delicious food) until I am better.
- I respect my body for doing its best under difficult circumstances, and I love it.

You may have more negative attitudes to add to the first list, and I hope you will have many more positive attitudes which you will decide to add to the second list. But remember, nothing happens until you make it happen, and the first way to implement such a plan is to write it down, and then practise it until it is a part of your thought pattern. Only then will you make it happen. How about starting right now, by scribbling at the end of these lists your negative attitudes (and make an immediate effort to realise they are there, and banish them), and your positive ones? Each time you feel negative about your body, or feel as though you are unhappy about your eating patterns, return to these lists and activate positive attitudes! It is as simple as that, if you practise.

DR DORA: How do people eat when stressed?

People tend to change their eating habits when they are stressed. One interesting study monitored people's diets and stress levels over a six-month period. During high workload periods, all of the subjects ate more saturated fat and sugar. Even in people who were usually restrained eaters, there was a tendency to binge when stress levels were high.[1] This implies that ongoing stress can adversely affect eating patterns in people who are usually healthy eaters.

Cravings and bingeing

Now that you understand how your body works, I hope you will listen to its needs with more understanding and knowledgeable ears. If you crave something, what can it mean?

If you crave sweet things:

It is usually a signal that your blood sugar levels have changed. The brain remembers that the last time a sweet thing was eaten, it was also effective in returning the sugar level back to normal, so the remembered link returns as a need for sweet things. These are often high GI foods, and so without knowing, the body has already learnt what it needs to rectify the situation, and what it tasted like. Clever, isn't it?

Your blood sugar level may be low, because you have not eaten for a while; you may have eaten a low GI carbohydrate at the last meal, which only gave you a short-acting burst of energy and which has already 'run out'; or you may simply not have eaten enough at the last meal. Eat something sweet, and then when you feel better, think about why it may have happened, and try not to make that mistake again.

You may have hormonal or chemical changes which have caused your sugar levels to drop: for instance a bout of nerves or stress, ongoing anxiety or depression. Perhaps you are pre-menstrual or going through menopause? Again, satisfy the need, and then deal with the underlying problem. If it is as simple as comfort-eating, then get some psychological advice from a professional about why this is happening, and keep listening to your body until your psychology is back to normal again. It will tell you when it is well – usually by stopping sending urgent 'need' messages – unless, of course, they are perfectly normal, such as the good old-fashioned hunger message when the petrol has run out!

Sometimes your blood sugar level may be fine, but your body still craves sweet things. This may be an indication of a 'faulty' serotonin function, and your body is simply trying to self-medicate that serotonin back to normal function again. Stay away from sweet things? No! Just understand that it may signal the need for an assessment with a psychiatrist, so that your serotonin levels can be returned to normal. Then you will naturally notice that those signals disappear as you get better. You should never consciously have to ignore them.

If you crave bread, potatoes (and potato crisps), cakes and croissants:

It may indicate the same problem: that your sugar levels need to be altered because they have dropped, or that your serotonin may need a boost. Remember that these are all high GI carbohydrates which will increase the blood sugar levels rapidly, thereby attaining the desired effect immediately. For many people with no mental or physical disorders, this job is done effectively, and the body's self-medication abilities have proved successful. However, the real problem may lie in three main areas:

- anxiety and depression
- insulin resistance
- obesity or fat gain.

In patients with anxiety or depression, the increase in sugar levels initiates a rise in the 'storage' chemical, insulin. This returns the sugar levels back to normal, but it is accompanied by a continual presence of the fight-or-flight chemicals, which serve to lower the sugar levels even further. This causes a rebound hypoglycaemia, which causes the blood sugar level to drop even further below normal. Clearly, this change is due to the physical abnormality, and not the food! When this 'overshoot' occurs, one experiences further depressive symptoms such as lethargy, anxiety, irritability, mood swings and more cravings, to try and aid the blood sugar level back to normal again. This is why some people mistakenly believe it to be a 'sugar addiction', when it is merely the body's way of repeatedly trying to rectify a symptom of an underlying and actually unrelated condition. Removing carbohydrates and sugars is simply removing a catalyst to a symptom, without recognising that there is an entirely different problem which needs to be dealt with. What's more, in persistent anxiety and clinical depression, cortisol is usually produced in excess. This leads directly to insulin resistance, and thus immediate storage of any fat that is eaten, thereby inducing fat gain.

Patients with insulin resistance release large amounts of insulin with each carbohydrate meal, because a normal amount of insulin would not be effective (the body cannot 'hear' insulin well enough). This also leads to a reactive hypoglycaemia, with each meal (especially the high GI carbohydrates) producing a blood sugar increase, followed by a dramatic sugar decrease, often below normal. These patients should take note of what types of carbohydrates they are eating, and how their bodies react. If the above scenario is the case, insulin levels should be checked and treated, and then the problem can be rectified. Until that time, however, control of sugar levels should be effected by sticking to the low GI carbohydrates only. This reduces the amount of insulin needing to be produced, and also maintains a more stable blood sugar level, reducing the potential for reactive hypoglycaemia. Remember that insulin is the storage chemical, and so the more insulin that the body produces, the more fats hidden in the food we eat will be stored, too. So, also removing dietary fats while supplementing with essential fatty acids will minimise this effectively, until such time as the insulin problem has been recified.

This is why people think that sweet things are fattening. Many sweet things are high GI carbohydrates, thereby stimulating the production of insulin. But remember that carbohydrates cannot make you fat. It is those hidden fats in those high GI foods which are stored immediately with so much insulin present storing everything it can! It is not the carbohydrates in the bread, cake and potatoes that are fattening for insulin-resistant patients, it is the paté, oil and butter eaten with those carbohydrates that are stored by the insulin. The clever way to deal with this is to:

- understand why the body is wanting these foods (self-medicating a problem which you ought to start addressing)
- satisfy the body's needs with whatever it wants: sweet things and high GI carbohydrates with no fats in them
- eat high GI carbohydrates with low GI carbohydrates, to maintain a steady sugar level, thereby 'safely' satisfying the craving
- recognise that there is a problem, and start concentrating on eating low GI carbohydrates to control the problem while you are sorting it out.

Never ignore a craving. Satisfy it, and then try to understand why it happened in the first place.

This may be a reason why many people binge. Think about what a binge actually is: it is an overwhelming desire to satisfy an overwhelming need. And what might cause this? The psychological and physical effects of depriving the body of what it needs, whether that be serotonin, energy, higher sugar levels or really good flavour. It is clear that the reasons for this litany of deprivations are depression and anxiety, calorie restriction, hunger and self-admonishment with bland, 'diet' foods. The answers are simple:

- satisfy the need, and eat until you feel better, no matter how much that is
- ensure that your food contains little or no fat (this provides the 'safety net' for bingeing: you won't gain fat if there are no fats present)
- deal with the problems, seek professional help for depression
- never calorie restrict again, never be hungry again, and eat good food!

If these rules are followed the patient will, with surprise and delight, reduce the binge-episodes dramatically without even trying, and never again feel such an urgent drive for excess.

So, with no further ado, I will end with my favourite motto:

Eat, drink and be merry!

13

PSYCHIATRIC THERAPY OF DEPRESSION, BULIMIA AND ANOREXIA

Dr Dora Wynchank

Psychiatric treatment of major depression

A historical view

We have discussed the definition of depression, what causes it and how it is diagnosed. Now let us focus on psychiatric treatment strategies. These days, we take it for granted that depression is treatable; but a glance at the history of medicine reminds us that effective, safe, tailor-made treatments are a recent phenomenon.

We start our historical journey in South America, where for centuries people have chewed the leaves of the coca plant to lift mood. Today, we recognise that the drug cocaine is extracted from this plant. Cocaine is known to lift mood and energy levels, and to decrease appetite. Until fairly recently, some respected specialists advocated the use of cocaine in the treatment of depression. In the last century, Freud, the founder of psychoanalysis, suggested that cocaine was a good treatment option in depression. Modern research has discredited cocaine as an effective antidepressant because it is addictive and does not elevate mood in a long-lasting way. Cocaine has been used recreationally as an illegal drug of abuse since the 1970s.

Another brave recommendation of 19th century psychiatrists was the use of hashish and coffee as treatment strategies for mood problems. Not surprisingly, these recommendations did not last long! Early treatments like these were bound to fail because at the time, there was no clear understanding of the neurotransmitter basis of the depression. The treatments were very much 'hit and miss'. Only in the last 50 years, as the underlying chemistry of depression has been unravelled, have effective treatments been made available.

The treatment of depression is basically divided into three areas:

- medication
- psychotherapy
- other (such as ECT or electroconvulsive therapy).

Medication

In most cases, a major depressive episode is treated with an antide-pressant medication for six months to two years. The combination of medication and psychotherapy works best. Often, drug treatment runs for longer than two years. There has been an explosion of treatments available in the last 20 years. Let's examine the types of antidepressants that are available today.

Monoamine oxidase inhibitors (MAOIs)

Discovery of the medical treatments for depression occurred about 50 years ago, and quite by chance. A breakthrough in the treatment of depression came in the early 1950s, when a new antibiotic for tuberculosis was being studied. Researchers found that patients on it became euphoric! This accident led to the first class of antidepressant ever discovered. The name of the class is a mouthful: the monoamine oxidase inhibitors (MAOIs). These drugs paralyse the enzyme (called MAO) that 'eats up' free serotonin and adrenaline, making more neurotransmitter available in the brain.

While these drugs are as effective as any newer antidepressant, they have serious side-effects. The main one is the 'cheese reaction'. MAOIs paralyse two forms of the MAO enzyme: type A and type B. Only type A destroys serotonin and adrenaline. Type B breaks down tyramine, an amino acid that causes an elevation of blood pressure. If both enzyme subtypes (A and B) are permanently paralysed by the antidepressant, then very high levels of tyramine accumulate which causes a danger-ously high blood pressure. Imagine the sorts of food you would have at a cocktail party: red wine, caviar, avocados, olives, cured meats, yeast products and cheese. These foods are all rich in tyramine. If tyramine-containing foods are eaten by someone on a MAOI, the tyramine cannot be broken down because the enzyme is paralysed. This results in the tyramine accumulating and causing high blood pressure, stroke or even death. For this reason, people taking MAOIs must stick to a special diet which excludes tyramine. Dietary restrictions are not easy to follow, so as a result, the MAOIs are only used as a last resort in the treatment of depression. There are some people who have an excellent response to these drugs and are faithful to the diet. They do well on the MAOIs.

Today, only one of these drugs is used – tranylcypromine (Parnate®). Other side effects of the MAOIs include:

- insomnia and agitation
- drop in blood pressure when standing
- sexual dysfunction.

Tricyclics

The next class of antidepressant to be discovered in the 1950s (also quite by accident) was the tricyclics. These are still used today. They are as effective as the newer antidepressants, but they have serious side-effects and are lethal in overdose. This makes them risky to use in the suicidally depressed patient. A core symptom of depression is suicidality: imagine the problems in giving a treatment where a week's supply could cause death by overdose!

Not all patients experience side-effects. However, tricyclics have more side-effects than other, newer antidepressants. Some of these disappear over time; some persist. Common side-effects of the tricyclics are:

- dry mouth
- blurred vision
- constipation
- tiredness
- weight gain
- sexual problems for both men and women, such as difficulty reaching orgasm.

The elderly are at risk for:

- low blood pressure
- effects on the heart, such as irregular heart beat, especially if there is an underlying cardiac problem
- difficulty urinating.

To prevent severe side-effects, a patient should be started on a low dose of a tricyclic. The dose is gradually increased. When stopping a tricyclic antidepressant, the patient must be weaned off slowly, to prevent a withdrawal reaction of:

- headache
- nausea
- diarrhoea
- restlessness.

Examples of the older tricyclics are imipramine, clomipramine and amitriptyline. Newer tricyclics, such as lofepramine, have fewer side-effects and are safe in overdose.

Selective Serotonin Reuptake Inhibitors (SSRIs)

Since the 1970s, when the neurotransmitter basis of depression began to be understood, antidepressants that increased the availability of serotonin have been developed. Today, five SSRIs are available:

- Citalopram (Cipramil®)
- Fluoxetine (Prozac®)
- Fluvoxamine (Luvox®)
- Paroxetine (Aropax®)
- Sertraline (Zoloft®).

The SSRIs have definite advantages compared to the tricyclics, although they are equally effective. With the SSRIs, side-effects tend to be milder and fewer. For this reason, it is often possible to start a patient on the total daily dose from day one. They are also safe in overdose. Although all five SSRIs share a common mechanism of action and are equally effective, they have different side-effect profiles. They tend to be well tolerated in the elderly. They are also useful for the treatment of depression associated with anxiety, as well as for specific anxiety disorders (such as panic attacks).

As a group, SSRIs share several side-effects which tend to disappear over the first 10 days:

- nausea and diarrhoea
- headache
- agitation (when starting the medication)
- sexual side-effects: difficulty achieving orgasm for women; delayed ejaculation for men. Occasionally, decreased sex drive occurs.

Other types of antidepressants

- **Mirtazapine (Remeron®):** Mirtazapine has a complex mechanism of action in that it increases the availability of both adrenaline and serotonin, but it also blocks two types of serotonin receptor. These receptors are 'baddies': when they are stimulated, they cause some of the side-effects seen with serotonergic antidepressants such as disturbed sleep, nausea and sexual dysfunction. When the 'baddies' are blocked, they are unable to preduce these side-effects. Side-effects that are caused by mirtazapine include sleepiness, increased appetite, weight gain and dry mouth.

- **Moclobemide (Aurorix®):** This antidepressant is a refined form of MAOI: it only inhibits the A form of the enzyme and it does not affect the enzyme permanently. There is no effect on tyramine and therefore no need for a special diet. Common side effects include insomnia, dizziness, headache and restlessness.
- **Nefazodone (Serzone®):** This antidepressant acts like an SSRI but also blocks one of the serotonin receptors. It also has an effect on adrenaline, increasing its availability in the brain. Side-effects include nausea, dizziness, dry mouth and tiredness. There is less insomnia and fewer sexual side-effects in patients treated with nefazodone.
- **Venlafaxine (Efexor®):** This antidepressant works by increasing the availability of both adrenaline and serotonin in the brain. Side-effects are similar to those found with the SSRIs: nausea, headache, dry mouth, insomnia and sexual dysfunction. Venlafaxine is available in a slow-release preparation, which has milder side-effects.

This is a bewildering list of medications; and there are new ones being developed all the time. Despite the choice and variety of antidepressants available today, the 'ideal' antidepressant has not yet been synthesised. The perfect antidepressant would work immediately, not interact with other medicines and have no side-effects. We've got a way to go!

Several points hold true for all antidepressants:
- They are all equally effective.
- They are all non-addictive.
- There are no long-term changes in personality after years of taking antidepressants.
- They all work in about 70% of people.
- They all take two to six weeks to lift depression (at an adequate dose).
- They all have side-effects; but the side-effect profiles differ.
- Not all people experience side-effects on antidepressants.

Psychotherapy in depression

A discussion of the psychological treatments of depression would require a book on its own! There are many schools of psychotherapy and each has a different approach for the treatment of depression. In most cases, a combination of medication and individual psychotherapy works best in treating depression. In some cases, family or marital therapy may be required.

Other forms of treatment:

Electroconvulsive therapy (ECT)

Anyone who has seen the film 'One flew over the cuckoo's nest' will be horrified that ECT is still used as a therapy for depression. While it is true that ECT used to be administered without anaesthetic and under terrible conditions, we know today that it is one of the safest and most effective treatments available in psychiatry. Unfortunately, misconceptions linger on, partly because of inflammatory articles in the lay press.

The history of inducing seizures to treat mental illness dates from the 1930s, when two Italian researchers used it to treat schizophrenia. ECT has raised considerable controversy since then and is no longer used to treat schizophrenia. Much research has proven that when correctly chosen for the treatment of severe depression, it is an excellent therapy. Today, ECT is administered under controlled circumstances; usually in an operating theatre. The procedure occurs under general anaesthetic, with monitoring of heart and lung function as well as complete muscle relaxation. It only takes a few minutes. During the treatment, a small electrical current is sent to the brain. This current produces a seizure that affects the entire brain, including the centres controlling mood, appetite and sleep. The seizure itself lasts about 25 seconds. It is usually given three times a week for two to three weeks (a total of six to nine treatments). ECT is very safe: the death rate with ECT is lower than that of childbirth. It does not cause brain trauma or any structural damage to the nervous system.

There are side-effects associated with ECT; although not everyone experiences them. The main one is memory loss. Forgetfulness occurs after a few treatments and may last up to several months. However, within six months, most people have completely recovered their memories. The one time period that remains blurred is the few weeks during which the ECT was given. After the course of ECT, there is no ongoing problem with laying down new memory. Occasionally, after ECT, people transiently forget things from the past (for example: the route to get to work). These memories are not permanently lost: once the person is reminded, the memory is retrieved and never forgotten again. Of course, memory problems are a defining feature of depression; so it is difficult to untangle what belongs to the depression and what to the treatment.

Another side effect of ECT is headache and confusion for about 20 minutes after the treatment.

The main advantage that ECT holds over traditional antidepressants is that it works immediately. It can be useful in a severely depressed and suicidal person where one cannot wait the six weeks necessary for an antidepressant to kick in. It is also an extremely safe treatment, especially in pregnancy. We use ECT in psychotic depression (where the person has completely lost touch with reality).

Generally, ECT is not used as a first line treatment of depression. Unfortunately, its effects are short-lived. Once the treatments are over, there is no protection against developing a future depressive episode. The patient is either started on an antidepressant or given 'maintenance ECT': one treatment every month, to prevent recurrence.

We definitely know that ECT works – but how? This is a fascinating area of study. We do not have all the answers yet. It appears that ECT has an effect on various neurotransmitters and their receptors. Chemical messengers in the brain are altered in a very similar way to what happens after a person has been on an antidepressant for several weeks. There may also be a change in blood flow in the brain.

Light therapy

Believe it or not, there are some forms of depression that occur in the northern hemisphere winter, at times of perpetual darkness. People suffering from this disorder tend to get depressed every year, at a specific season, usually winter. Where there is a seasonal component to depression, improvement may occur with exposure to light. Bright white artificial light is used for about half an hour in the mornings, immediately after waking. A shift in mood is seen within three to four days; usually by two weeks there is total improvement. The 'side-effects' of light therapy are headache, eyestrain, irritability and insomnia.

The 'holistic' approach to treatment

Treatment of depression should be as multifaceted as possible. Don't stop at medication and psychotherapy! Other important areas to address are exercise, diet and relaxation. Support groups can play an important role for both family members and depressives themselves. They provide education and lobby for those suffering from the disorder. Education is essential. Understand the illness; remove the stigma.

How to treat depression: the acute phase

- The doctor you visit should take a thorough history and do an examination. As we have discussed, medical problems, drugs or alcohol can all cause depression. These should be excluded before a diagnosis of major depression is made.

- For a first episode of major depression, in the acute phase of treatment, an antidepressant is indicated. Be aware of what to expect in terms of side-effects. Up to 15% of people stop taking their treatment within the first three weeks. This is usually because they were not warned about the initial side-effects. After the first day of nausea, they imagine that it will continue permanently!
- Be aware that all antidepressants take between two and six weeks to work, at a therapeutic dose. Don't expect miracles early on! In the first week, certain antidepressants do help lower anxiety levels, but the disturbed physical functions of depression take longer to clear.
- Symptoms of depression do not lift simultaneously. The improvement tends to occur in a staggered way. For example, anxiety often lifts first, followed by an improvement in appetite. In the second week, concentration and memory may become sharper. By the third week, sleep is more restful and energy levels increase. All this time, mood is still down, with feelings of hopelessness and thoughts of death. Finally, in the fifth week, mood improves.
- Side-effects should be monitored. If they are incapacitating, the medication should be stopped and another antidepressant started.
- If there is an inadequate response after the first four weeks of treatment, the dose of the antidepressant may be increased.
- A failed trial of an antidepressant suggests that another antidepressant, usually from a different class, is indicated. In the case of a partial response, other medications may be used to boost the action of the antidepressant. This process is called augmentation.

How to treat depression: the continuation phase

Once the episode of depression has been successfully treated, you enter the continuation phase of treatment. Understand that a first episode of depression should be treated for between six months and two years. If medication is stopped sooner, there is a high chance of relapse. During the continuation phase, psychotherapy is often indicated. We know that depression tends to be a chronic, even lifelong illness. Even after one has recovered fully from one episode, there is a high chance of relapse. About two-thirds of people who have one major depressive episode will have another, usually in the next two years. If one has had three serious, life-threatening episodes of depression, treatment should probably continue for life.

How to treat depression: the maintenance phase

If this is not the first episode, longer-term maintenance treatment may be necessary. The more frequent and severe the previous episodes, the more important it is to continue with treatment. The dose of the maintenance phase treatment should be the same as the dose that got you well. There is no evidence that the effects of antidepressants 'wear off' over time. The same dose should be used for as long as treatment continues – for some people, this may be for life.

Stopping your antidepressant

There are certain rules to follow when discontinuing antidepressants.

- Most of the newer antidepressants do not cause withdrawal symptoms when they are stopped. However, some people believe that all antidepressants should be tapered off slowly, to prevent relapse.
- If you stop your antidepressant, do it with your doctor's knowledge.
- You should be aware of the early warning bells of a new depressive episode. For every person, these are different. Learn how to recognise a new episode early on, so it can be nipped in the bud. If a particular antidepressant previously worked for you, it makes sense to use it again.

Is depression overtreated?

You have almost certainly read, in sensationalist magazines, of an explosion in antidepressant prescribing. Is it accurate to call Prozac® the drug of the nineties? However convincing they sound, these statements are grossly incorrect. All of the scientific research into depression has consistently shown that it is both underrecognised and undertreated. Why? There are two basic reasons for this which we will explore in some detail.

Depressives do not seek help

- In a large American community study, only two-thirds of people with major depression sought treatment.[1]
- Even when they have been suffering for months, depressives tend to under-use medical facilities. The same study found that after a year of being depressed, only 20% sought professional help.[2]
- Other studies have shown that in the early 1990s, only 2-25% of depressives in the community sought help.[3-5]

Doctors miss the diagnosis

- About 10 years ago, doctors were much less informed about depression. They tended to miss the diagnosis, even when all of the signs and symptoms were there. Overall, only 10% of patients with major depression received an adequate dose of an antidepressant for an adequate period of time.[6] This meant that 90% of people either slipped through the net completely or were undertreated!

- Later on in the 1990s, when patients did get to a primary health care clinic, another study showed that doctors performed better. They correctly identified two-thirds of depressed cases. Over 50% of these depressed patients were given antidepressants.[7] Diagnostic skill was not yet ideal, but it was improving!

- Sadly, psychiatrists did not do better than family doctors when it came to treating depressed people.[8] Many patients were started on treatment by their psychiatrists, but then they were lost to follow-up.

These studies examine American populations of patients and doctors. We can expect that in countries where there is less access to clinics and health care facilities, even fewer patients get treatment. Doctors' training is also at fault: many family doctors are poorly educated about depression.

Why bother to treat depression?

Treating depression is expensive and time-consuming: is it really necessary? The emphatic answer is yes! Depression kills and depression costs more if untreated – both economically and in terms of human suffering. We have emphasised many times in this book that depression is not a benign illness. Untreated depression affects daily functioning in over half of patients.[9] Depressed patients experience a poor quality of life that is worse than in many other common medical conditions, such as heart disease, arthritis and kidney disease.[10] This may be because it is a 'mental illness' affecting emotions, relationships and the ability to take pleasure in one's surroundings.

Work productivity falls in depressed people, which is very costly to employers.[11] In fact, in America, depression has been estimated to cost $44 billion per year![12,13] This is a vast sum. The majority of the cost is due to reduced productivity of depressed workers, excessive absenteeism and death due to suicide; admitting people to hospital and treating them with medication accounts for a smaller proportion of the sum.

Another complication of untreated depression is that it rarely exists alone. Depressed people tend to have more than one problem that needs treatment. So, in targeting and treating the depression, one may also be able to treat a co-existing anxiety or substance abuse problem as well as any physical problem such as cancer. The outcome is much worse for the depressed person with other psychiatric diagnoses in addition to depression.

Psychiatric treatment of anorexia nervosa

Everyone agrees that it is difficult to treat anorexia. The treatment outcome is poor.

- Very occasionally, anorexics do not require treatment – they may recover spontaneously.
- About one quarter recover after a number of treatments. About 10% fluctuate: they may get better and then worse, but all in all they remain unchanged.
- About one fifth of anorexics progress to develop bulimia nervosa.
- For 20%, the illness remains a lifelong problem.
- A small proportion seems immune to treatment. They gradually deteriorate until they die from the effects of starvation. The mortality rate in anorexia is between 5 and 10%. Patients who do poorly have lower weights, have failed treatment programmes, vomit to lose weight, have dysfunctional family backgrounds and are married.[14]

In general, anorexia is a complicated illness to treat, given the combination of medical and psychiatric factors that co-exist.

When treating an anorexic, the first question is: should she be admitted to hospital? The degree to which she is underweight determines whether or not she is admitted. Generally, when the anorexic is 20% underweight, she needs admission.

Specialised psychiatric units treat anorexics over a period of several months. A combination of treatments is required. Medical interventions reverse the damage done to the body by starvation. Sometimes, a hospital admission can be life-saving. There are two main aims of admission to hospital:

- stopping weight loss with eventual weight gain
- reverting to normal eating patterns.

The patient is placed on an eating programme with structured meal times. Weight is gained at about 1 kg per week. Ideally, the patient should reach a target weight of 90% of what is acceptable for her weight and height. In addition, behavioural programmes reward weight gain with privileges.

Psychotherapy is not particularly helpful in the early stages, when anorexics are still extremely underweight. Prolonged starvation makes people irrational; it also affects mood and behaviour.[15] Often, anorexics are poorly motivated for therapy. Later on, individual therapy certainly plays a role. Family and group therapy are often both necessary. Educating the patient and the family about the disorder is essential.

Many anorexics resist hospitalisation. They do not see that they are underweight and deny the problem.

Medication in anorexia nervosa

Many years ago, the main medical treatment of anorexia was an antipsychotic drug in a low dose. At times, anorexics seem to lose touch with reality: they 'see' bags of fat hanging off an emaciated frame; they stubbornly refuse to eat even though they look skeletal. These drugs do have a place in the treatment of very agitated anorexics. Even though it may seem intuitively correct to treat anorexics with antipsychotics, very little research substantiates their use. The SSRIs may improve depressed mood, obsessive thinking and refusal to gain weight. However, this remains controversial, as depression tends to lift as weight is gained anyway. Underweight patients are more prone to side-effects of medication.

Psychiatric treatment of bulimia nervosa

Improvement in bulimics on treatment is often dramatic and recovery is the rule. As a group, bulimics do better with treatment than anorexics.

- Half of all bulimics on treatment recover fully.
- Forty per cent improve, with some symptoms persisting.
- Only 10% do not respond to treatment and have a severe, chronic course.[16] A predictor for poor outcome is personality structure.

Most bulimics are best treated as outpatients, attending an eating disorders clinic or a therapist specialising in the disorder. Admission to hospital is only necessary when the usual clinic treatment fails. If there is severe drug or alcohol abuse or the bulimic has an additional problem of suicidal depression, admission should be considered.[17] Occasionally, the medical condition of the bulimic deteriorates to the point where admission is necessary. Hospital admissions are usually for several weeks.

Any medical problem should be investigated and treated. Laxatives should be stopped. Drinking six to eight glasses of water per day is encouraged to improve bowel function. Exercise also helps.

Psychotherapy is an important component of the treatment of bulimia. The form of psychotherapy best studied is cognitive behavioural therapy (CBT). At least 26 studies have compared CBT to other forms of psychotherapy. The results of these studies show that it does well as a treatment modality. After CBT, bingeing episodes decrease by 60% and purging decreases by 45%. During CBT, bulimics are challenged in the way they think and behave. The therapy has several components.

- Education is a common starting point in therapy.
- Self-monitoring follows. Bulimics are encouraged to keep diaries of their feelings, urges to binge and behaviours.[18] Reviewing the diary with a therapist works well in identifying what precipitates a binge. During the course of therapy, progress may be monitored.
- Illogical thoughts about weight, shape and body image are challenged in therapy.
- Nutritional counselling helps the patient eat in a balanced and regular way, even after the therapy is over.

Self-help groups like Overeaters Anonymous may help to prevent relapse. Family therapy may be necessary.

Medication in bulimia nervosa

There is strong evidence that antidepressants work in bulimia. SSRIs in high doses reduce binging and vomiting behaviours by up to a third.[19] Attitude towards weight and shape also changes when these medications are used. Antidepressants work in bulimia, whether or not the patient is depressed. A combination of CBT and antidepressant works better than either therapy alone.

Depression occurs in 5% of bulimics. Where it is present, it should be treated. The most important message in the treatment of bulimia is that it responds well to treatment, which should be started as soon as possible.

REFERENCES

1. The stigma attached to clinical depression

1. Coombe G, 1834. *Elements of phrenology.* MA, Marsh, Capen and Lyon
2. Hoyersten JG, 1996. Som besatt! Noen historiske, psykiatriske og aktuelle momenter ved demonbesettelse. (Possessed! Some historical, psychiatric and current moments of demonic possession). *Tidsskrift for den Norske Laegeforening* 116:30, 3602-6
3. Mathew VM *et al*, 1991. Attempted suicide and the lunar cycle. *Psychological Reports* 68:3 (Pt 1), 927-30
4. Gorvin JJ, Roberts MS, 1994. Lunar phases and psychiatric hospital admissions. *Psychological Reports* 75:3 (Pt 2), 1435-40
5. Templer DI, Veleber DM, 1980. The moon and madness: a comprehensive perspective. *Journal of Clinical Psychology* 36:4, 865-8
6. Sands JM, Miller LE, 1991. Effects of moon phase and other temporal variables on absenteeism. *Psychological Reports* 69:3 (Pt 1), 959-62
7. Mathew VM *et al*, 1991, *op cit.*
8. Kendell RE, Zealley AK (eds), 1988. *Companion to psychiatric studies* (4th ed). Churchill Livingstone
9. Freeman H, 1996. 250 Jahre englische Psychiatrie (250 years of English psychiatry). *Fortschritte der Neurologie Psychiatrie* 64:8, 320-26
10. Gelder MG, 1996. Biological psychiatry in perspective. *British Medical Bulletin* 52:3, 401-7
11. Lion JR (ed), 1981. *Personality disorders: diagnosis and management* (2nd ed). Williams & Wilkins, Baltimore
12. American Psychiatric Association, 1994. *Diagnostic and Statistical Manual of Mental Disorders* (4th ed). Washington, DC: APA
13. Cloninger RC, Svrakic DM, Przybeck TR, 1993. A psychobiological model of temperament and character. *Archives of General Psychiatry* 50
14. Keller MB *et al*, !982. Treatment received by depressed patients. *Journal of the American Medical Association* 248:15, 1848-55
15. Keller MB *et al*, 1992. Time to recovery, chronicity and levels of psychopathology in major depression: A 5 year prospective follow-up of 431 subjects. *Archives of General Psychiatry* 49, 809-16
16. Ader R, Cohen N, 1975. Behaviourally conditioned immunosuppression. *Psychosomatic Medicine* 37:4, 333-40
17. Folkman S, Lazarus RS, 1985. If it changes it must be a process: study of emotion and coping during three stages of a college examination. *Journal of Personality and Social Psychology* 48, 150-70

18. Kiecolt-Glaser JK, Glaser R, 1988. Psychological influences on immunity: Making sense of the relationship between stressful life events and health. *Advances in Experimental Medicine and Biology* 245, 237
19. Dorian B, Garfinkel PE, 1987. Stress, immunity and illness – a review. *Psychological Medicine* 17, 393-407
20. Dorian B, Garfinkel PE, Brown G et al, 1982. Aberrations in lymphocyte subpopulation and function during psychological stress. *Clinical and Experimental Immunology* 50, 132-138
21. Dorian B, Garfinkel PE, 1987, op cit.
22. Hinkle LE, 1973. The concept of 'stress' in the biological and social sciences. *Science, Medicine and Man* 1, 3148

2. What is stress?

1. Lazarus RS, 1966. *Psychological stress and the coping process*. McGraw-Hill, New York
2. Holmes T, 1978. Life situations, emotions and disease. *Psychosomatic Medicine* 19, 747
3. Solomon GF, 1987. Psychoneuroimmunology: interactions between central nervous system and immune system. *Journal of Neuroscience Research* 18, 1
4. Ader R, Cohen N, Felten D, 1987. Brain, behaviour, and immunity. *Brain, Behaviour and Immunity* 1, 1
5. Brown GW, Harris T, 1978. *Social origins of depression*. Tavistock Publications, London
6. Paykel ES, Myers JK, Dienelt MN et al, 1969. Life event and depression: a controlled study. *Archives of General Psychiatry* 21, 753
7. Surtees PG et al, 1986. Life events and the onset of affective disorder: a longitudinal general population study. *Journal of Affective Disorders* 10, 37
8. Surtees PG, Sashidharan SP, 1986. Psychiatric morbidity in two matched community samples: a comparison of rates and risks in Edinburgh and St Louis. *Journal of Affective Disorders* 10, 101
9. Brenner JD et al, 1997. MRI-based measurement of hippocampal volume in post-traumatic stress disorder. *Biological Psychiatry* 41, 23-32
10. American Psychiatric Association, 1994. *Diagnostic and Statistical Manual of Mental Disorders* (4th ed). Washington, DC: APA
11. *Ibid*
12. Realini JP, Katerndahl DA, 1991. *Threshold for seeking care*. Presented at the North American Primary Care Research Group Meeting, May 23-25, 1991, Quebec City, Canada
13. Wulsin LR, Hillard JR, Geier P, 1988. Screening emergency room patients with atypical chest pain for depression and panic disorder. *International Journal of Psychiatry and Medicine* 18, 315-23
14. Beitman BD, Lambert JW, Mukerji V, 1987. Panic disorder in patients with angiographically normal coronary arteries. *Psychosomatics* 28, 480-84
15. Otto MW, Pollack MH. Treatment strategies for panic disorder: a debate. *Harvard Review of Pychiatry* 2, 166-70
16. Beck AAT, 1988. Cognitive approaches to panic disorder: theory and therapy. In: Rachman S, Maser JD (eds), *Panic: Psychological Perspectives*. Hillsdale; NJ: Lawrence Arlbaum Associates, 91-109
17. American Psychiatric Association, 1980. *Diagnostic and Statistical Manual of Mental Disorders* (3rd ed). Washington DC: APA
18. Van Putten T, Emory WM, 1973. Traumatic neurosis in Vietnam returnees: a forgotten diagnosis. *Archives of General Psychiatry* 29, 695-98

19. Helzer JE, Robins LN, McEvoy L, 1987. Posttraumatic stress disorder in the general population. *New England Journal of Medicine* 317, 1630-34
20. Hryvniak M, Rosse R, 1989. Concurrent psychiatric illness in inpatients with PTSD. *Military Medicine* 154, 399-401

3. What is clinical depression?

1. Leon AC, Klerman GL, Wickramaratne P, 1993. Continuing female predominance in depressive illness. *American Journal of Public Health* 83:5, 754-57
2. Regier DA, Boyd JH, Burke JD Jr et al, 1988. One-month prevalence of mental disorders in the United States. *Archives of General Psychiatry* 45, 977-86
3. Weissman MM, Olfson M, 1995. Depression in women: implications for health care research. *Science* 269, 799-801
4. Weissman MM, Klerman GL, 1977. Sex differences and the epidemiology of depression. *Archives of General Psychiatry* 34, 98-111
5. Weissman MM, Bland R, Joyce PR et al, 1993. Sex differences in rates of depression: cross-national perspectives. *Journal of Affective Disorders* 29, 77-84
6. Kessler RC, McGonagle KA, Swartz M *et al*, 1993. Sex and depression in the National Comorbidity Survey, I: lifetime prevalence, chronicity, and recurrence. *Journal of Affective Disorders* 29, 85-96
7. Kornstein SG, 1997. Gender differences in depression: implications for treatment. *Journal of Clinical Psychiatry* 58 (suppl 15), 12-18
8. Sikich L, Todd RD, 1988. Are the neurodevelopmental effects of gonadal hormones related to sex differences in psychiatric illnesses? *Psychiatric Development* 6:4, 277-309
9. Zlotnick C *et al*, 1996. Gender, type of treatment, dysfunctional attitudes, social support, life events, and depressive symptoms over naturalistic follow-up. *American Journal of Psychiatry* 153:8, 1021-27
10. Corney RH 1990. Sex differences in general practice attendance and help seeking for minor illness. *Psychosomatic Research* 34:5, 525-34
11. Sajatovic M, Vernon L, Semple W, 1997. Clinical characteristics and health resource use of men and women veterans with serious mental illness. *Psychiatric Services* 48:11, 1461-63
12. Friedman M, Thoresen CE, Gill JJ *et al*, 1982. Feasibility of altering type A behaviour pattern after myocardial infarction: Recurrent Coronary Prevention Project Study: Methods, baseline results, and preliminary findings. *Circulation* 66, 83
13. American Psychiatric Association, 1994. *Diagnostic and Statistical Manual of Mental Disorders* (4th ed). Washington, DC: APA
14. Thase ME, Simons AD, Reynolds CF, 1996. Abnormal electroencephalographic sleep profiles in major depression. *Archives of General Psychiatry* 53, 99-108
15. Twarog BM and Page IH, 1953. Serotonin content of some mammalian tissues and urine and method for its determination. *American Journal of Physiology* 175, 157-161
16. Reiman EM, Raichle ME, Robins E, 1989. Neuroanatomical correlates of a lactate induced anxiety attack. *Archives of General Psychiatry* 46, 493-500
17. Delgado PL, Miller HL, Salomon RM, 1993. Monoamines and the mechanism of antidepressant action: effects of catecholamine depletion on mood of patients treated with antidepressants. *Psychopharmacological Bulletin* 29, 389-396
18. Traskman L, Asberg M, Bertilsson L, Sjostrand L, 1981. Monoamine metabolites in CSF and suicidal behaviour. *Archives of General Psychiatry* 38, 631-636

19. Charney DS, Woods SW, Goodman WK, Heninger GR, 1987. Serotonin function in anxiety. II. Effects of the serotonin agonist MCPP in panic disorder patients and healthy subjects. *Psychopharmacology* 92, 14-24
20. Cloninger CR, 1990. Comorbidity of anxiety and depression. *Journal of Clinical Psychopharmacology* 10, 43S-6S
21. Rickels K, Schhweizer E, 1993. The treatment of generalised anxiety disorder in patients with depressive symtomatology. *Journal of Clinical Psychiatry* 54
22. Wittchen HU, Essau CA, Krieg JC, 1991. Anxiety disorders: similarities and differences of comorbidity in treated and untreated groups. *British Journal of Psychiatry* 159 (12, suppl), 23-33
23. Noyes RN Jr, 1991. Suicide and panic disorder: a review. *Journal of Affective Disorders* 22, 1-11
24. Clayton PJ, Grove WM, Coryell W, 1992. Follow-up and family study of anxious depression. *American Journal of Psychiatry* 149, 100-7
25. American Psychiatric Association, 1994, *op cit*
26. *Ibid*

4. The HPA axis

1. Mendelwicz J, Linkowski P, Brauman H, 1979. TSH responses to TRH in women with unipolar and bipolar depression. *Lancet* 2, 1079-80
2. Schilkrut R, Chandra O, Osswald M, 1975. Growth hormone during sleep and with thermal stimulation in depressed patients. *Neuropsychobiology* 1, 70-79
3. Plotsky PM, Owens MJ, Nemeroff CB, 1998. Psychoneuroendocrinology of depression. Hypothalamic-pituitary-adrenal axis. *Psychiatric Clinics of North America* 21:2, 293-307
4. Carpenter W, Bunney W, 1971. Adrenal cortical activity in depressive illness. *American Journal of Psychiatry* 128, 31
5. Carroll BJ, Curtis GC, Davies BM, 1976. Urinary free cortisol excretion in depression. *Journal of Psychological Medicine* 6, 43
6. Gibbons JL, McHugh PR, 1962. Plasma cortisol in depressive illness. *Journal of Psychiatric Research* 1, 162
7. Sachar EJ, Hellman L, Fukushima D, 1970. Cortisol production in depressive illness. *Archives of General Psychiatry* 23, 289
8. Carroll BJ, 1968. Pituitary adrenal function in depression. *Lancet* 1, 1373
9. Arato M, Banki CM, Bisette G, 1989. Elevated CSF CRF in suicide victims. *Biological Psychiatry* 25, 355
10. Kathol RG, Jaeckle RS, Lopez JF, Meller WH, 1989. Pathophysiology of HPA axis abnormalities in patients with Major Depression: an update. *American Journal of Psychiatry* 146, 3
11. Heim C, Nemeroff CB, 1999. The impact of early adverse experiences on brain systems involved in the pathophysiology of anxiety and affective disorders. *Biological Psychiatry* 1:46, 1509-22
12. Coplan JD et al, 1996. Persistent elevations of cerebrospinal fluid concentrations of corticotropin-releasing factor in adult nonhuman primates exposed to early life stressors: implications for the pathophysiology of mood and anxiety disorders. *Proceedings of the National Academy of Sciences of the USA* 93, 1619-23
13. Kaufman J et al, 1997. The corticotrophin-releasing hormone challenge in depressed abused, depressed nonabused, and normal control children. *Biological Psychiatry* 20, 669-79
14. Aborelius L, Owens MJ, Plotsky PM, Nemeroff CB, 1999. The role of corticotropin-releasing factor in depression and anxiety disorders. *Journal of Endocrinology* 160:1, 1-12

15. Finkelhor K, 1987. The sexual abuse of children: current research reviewed. *Psychiatry Annals* 17, 233-41
16. Herman JP, Adams D, Prewitt C, 1995. Regulatory changes in neuroendocrine stress-integrative circuitary produced by a variable stress paradigm. *Neuroendocrinology* 61, 180-90
17. Clarke JN, 1999. Chronic fatigue syndrome: gender differences in the search for legitimacy. *Australia and New Zealand Journal of Mental Health Nursing* 8:4, 123-33
18. Van der Steen WJ, 2000. Chronic fatigue syndrome: a matter of enzyme deficiencies? *Cancer Treatment Review* 54:5, 853-54
19. Lawrie SM et al, 2000. The difference in patterns of motor and cognitive function in chronic fatigue syndrome and severe depressive illness. *Psychological Medicine* 30:2, 433-42
20. Schmaling KB, Smith WR, Buchwald DS, 2000. Significant other responses are associated with fatigue and functional status among patients with chronic fatigue syndrome. *Psychosomatic Medicine* 62:3, 444-50
21. Werbach MR, 2000. Nutritional strategies for treating chronic fatigue syndrome. *Alternative Medicine Review* 5, 93-108
22. Price JR, Couper J, 2000. Cognitive behaviour therapy for adults with chronic fatigue syndrome. *Cochrane Database Systemic Review* 2, CD001027

5. Carbohydrates and serotonin

1. Wurtman J, Hefti F, Melamed E, 1980. Precursor contol of neurotransmitter synthesis. *Pharmacological Reviews* 32, 315-35
2. Sayegh R *et al*, 1995. The effect of a carbohydrate-rich beverage on mood, appetite, and cognitive function in women with prementstrual syndrome. *Obstetrics and Gynecology* 86:4, 520-28

6. Why is food the enemy?

1. Golay A, 2000. Similar weight loss with low-energy food combining or balanced diets. *International Journal of Obesity Related Metabolic Disorders* 24:4, 492-96
2. Green MW, Rogers PJ, 1995. Impaired cognitive functioning during spontaneous dieting. *Psychological Medicine* 25, 1003-10
3. National Institute of Diabetes and Digestive and Kidney Diseases, Bethesda, MD, USA, 2000. Overweight, obesity, and health risk. National Task Force on the Prevention and Treatment of Obesity. *Archives of Internal Medicine* 160:7, 898-904
4. World Health Organisation report on obesity, 1997
5. Dickerson LM, Carek PJ, 2000. Drug therapy for obesity. *American Family Physician* 61:7, 2131-38, 2143
6. Galtier-Dereure F, Boegner C, Bringer J, 2000. Obesity and pregnancy: complications and cost. *American Journal of Clinical Nutrition* 71 Suppl[5], 1242S-48S
7. Van Deth R, Vandereycken W, 2000. Food refusal and insanity: sitophobia and anorexia nervosa in Victorian asylums. *International Journal of Eating Disorders* 27:4, 390-404
8. Bemporad JR, 1996. Self-starvation through the ages: reflections on the pre-history of anorexia nervosa. *International Journal of Eating Disorders* 19:3, 217-37
9. Johnson SR, 1987. The epidemiology and social impact of premenstrual symptoms. *Clinical Obstetrics and Gynecology* 30, 369-384

10. Merikangas KR, Foeldenyl M, Angst J, 1993. The Zurich Study XIX. Patterns of menstrual disturbances in the community: results of the Zurich Cohort Study. *European Archives of Psychiatry and Clinical Neuroscience* 243, 23-32
11. Rivera-Tovar AD, Frank E, 1990. Late luteal phase dysphoric disorder in young women. *American Journal of Psychiatry* 147, 1634-36
12. Woods NF, Most FA, Dery GK, 1982. Prevalence of perimenstrual symptoms. *American Journal of Public Health* 71, 1257-64
13. Ramcharan S, Love EJ, Fick GH et al, 1992. The epidemiology of premenstrual symptoms in a population-based sample of 2650 urban women: attributable risk and risk factors. *Journal of Clinical Epidemiology* 45, 377-92
14. American Psychiatric Association, 1994. *Diagnostic and Statistical Manual of Mental Disorders* (DSM-IV) (4th ed) Washington
15. Wurtman J, Hefti F, Melamed E, 1980. Precursor contol of neurotransmitter synthesis. *Pharmacological Reviews* 32, 315-35
16. Sayegh R et al, 1995. The effect of a carbohydrate-rich beverage on mood, appetite, and cognitive function in women with premenstrual syndrome. *Obstetrics and Gynecology* 86:4 Pt 1, 520-28
17. Thys-Jacobs S, 2000. Micronutrients and the premenstrual syndrome: the case for calcium. *Journal of the American College of Nutrition* 19:2, 220-27

7. Food obsessions: how common are they?

1. American Psychiatric Association, 1994. *Diagnostic and Statistical Manual of Mental Disorders* (4th ed). Washington
2. Mussell MP et al, 1995. Onset of binge eating, dieting, obesity, and mood disorders among subjects seeking treatment for binge eating disorder. *International Journal of Eating Disorders* 17:4, 395-401
3. Tzischinsky O et al, 2000. Sleep-wake cycles in women with binge eating disorder. *International Journal of Eating Disorders* 27:1, 43-8
4. Kinzl JF et al, 1999. Binge eating disorder in females: a population-based investigation. *International Journal of Eating Disorders* 25:3, 287-92
5. Howard CE, Porzelius LK, 1999. The role of dieting in binge eating disorder: etiology and treatment implications. *Clinical Psychology Review* 19:1, 25-44
6. Grilo CM, Masheb RM , 2000. Onset of dieting vs binge eating in outpatients with binge eating disorder. *International Journal of Obesity Related Metabolic Disorders* 24:4, 404-9
7. Fairburn CG et al, 1998. Risk factors for binge eating disorder: a community-based, case-control study. *Arch ives of General Psychiatry* 55:5, 425-32
8. Kinzl JF et al, 1999, *op cit*
9. Mussell MP et al, 1995, *op cit*
10. Davis C, Claridge G, 1998. The eating disorders as addiction: a psychobiological perspective. *Addictive Behaviours* 23:4, 463-75
11. Bamber D, Cockerill IM, Carroll D, 2000. The pathological status of exercise dependence. *British Journal of Sports Medicine* 34:2, 125-32
12. Fernstrom J, Wurtman R, 1972. Brain serotonin content: increase following ingestion of carbohydrate diet. *Science* 173, 1023-25
13. Wurtman R, 1989. Carbohydrates and depression. *Scientific American* 68-75
14. Szczypka MS, Rainey MA, Palmiter RD, 2000. Dopamine is required for hyperphagia in Lepob/ob mice. *Nature Genetics* 25:1, 102-104

15. Guertin TL, 1999. Eating behaviour of bulimics, self-identified binge eaters, and non eating disordered individuals: what differentiates these populations? *Clinical Psychology Review* 19, 1-23
16. Schlundt DG et al, 1993. A sequential behavioural analysis of craving sweets in obese women. *Addictive Behaviours* 18, 67-80
17. Kaye WH *et al*, 1987. Reduced cerebrospinal fluid levels of immunoreactive pro-opiomelanocortin related peptides (including beta-endorphin) in anorexia nervosa. *Life Sciences* 41:18, 2147-55
18. Davis C, Claridge G, 1998. The eating disorders as addiction: a psychobiological perspective. *Addictive Behaviours* 23:4, 463-75
19. Marrazzi MA, et al, 1997. Endogenous codeine and morphine in anorexia and bulimia nervosa. *Life Sciences* 60:20, 1741-7
20. Gordon CM et al, 2000. Neuroanatomy of human appetitive function: A positron emission tomography investigation. *International Journal of Eating Disorders* 27:2, 163-71
21. Hirschberg AL, 1998. Hormonal regulation of appetite and food intake. *Annals of Medicine* 30:1, 7-20
22. Weltzin TE, Fernstrom MH, Kaye WH, 1994. Serotonin and bulimia nervosa. *Nutritional Review* 52:12, 399-408
23. Weltzin K, 1991. Serotonin activity in anorexia and bulimia. *Journal of Clinical Psychiatry* 52 (Suppl), 41-48
24. Leibowitz SF, Alexander JT, 1998. Hypothalamic serotonin in control of eating behavior, meal size, and body weight. *Biological Psychiatry* 44:9, 851-64

8. How calorie restricting leads to clinical depression.

1. Wurtman JJ, 1990. Carbohydrate craving. Relationship between carbohydrate intake and disorders of mood. *Drugs* 39 (Suppl) 3, 49-52
2. Mussell MP *et al*, 1995. Onset of binge eating, dieting, obesity and mood disorders among subjects seeking treatment for binge eating disorer. *International Journal of Eating Disorders* 174, 395-401
3. Wurtman J, Hefti F, Melamed E, 1980. Precursor contol of neurotransmitter synthesis. *Pharmacological Reviews* 32, 315-35
4 Knott VJ *et al*, 1999. The effect of acute tryptophan depletion and fenfluramine on quantitative EEG and mood in healthy male subjects. *Journal of Clinical Psychiatry* 60, 414-420
5. Young SN *et al*, 1985. Tryptophan depletion causes a rapid lowering of mood in normal males. *Psychopharmacology* 87, 173-77
6. Young SN *et al*, 1989. Biochemical aspects of tryptophan depletion in primates. *Psychopharmacology* 98, 508-11
7. Delgado PL *et al*, 1994. Serotonin and the neurobiology of depression: effects of tryptophan depletion in drug-free depressed patients. *Archives of General Psychiatry* 51:11, 865-74
8. Smith KA, Fairburn CG, Cowen PJ, 1997. Relapse of depression after rapid depletion of tryptophan. *Lancet* 349, 915-19
9. Asberg-Wistedt A *et al*, 1998. Serotonergic 'vulnerability' in affective disorder: a study of the tryptophan depletion test and relationships between peripheral and central serotonin indexes in citalopram-responders. *Acta Psychiatrica Scandinavia* 97, 374-80
10. Markus CF *et al*, 1998. Does carbohydrate-rich, protein-poor food prevent a deterioration of mood and cognitive performance of stress-prone subjects when subjected to a stressful task? *Appetite* 31:1, 49-65
11. Christensen L, Somers S, 1996. Comparison of nutrient intake among depressed and non-depressed individuals. *InternationalJournal of Eating Disorders* 20:1, 105-109

12. Laffel L, 1999. Ketone bodies: a review of physiology, pathophysiology and application of monitoring to diabetes. *Diabetes/Metabolism Reviews* 16:6, 412-26
13. Blundell JE, Cooling J, 1999. High-fat and low-fat (behavioural) phenotypes: biology or environment? Proceedings of the Nutrition Society 58:4, 773-77

9. How dieting can lead to an eating disorder

1. Vitiello B, Lederhendler I, 2000. Research on eating disorders: current status and future prospects. *Biological Psychiatry* 47:9, 777-86
2. Rodin J, Silberstein L, Striegel-Moore R, 1984. Women and weight: a normative discontent. In: Sonderegger TB (ed), *Psychology and gender: Nebraska symposium on motivation.* University of Nebraska Press, Lincoln
3. Holland AJ *et al*, 1984. Anorexia nervosa: a study of 34 twin pairs and one set of triplets. *British Journal of Psychiatry* 145, 414
4. Kaye WH *et al*, 2000. A search for susceptibility loci for anorexia nervosa: methods and sample description. *Biological Psychiatry* 47:9, 794-803
5. Minuchin S, Rosman B, Baker L, 1978. *Psychosomatic families: anorexia nervosa in context.* Cambridge, Massachusetts: Harvard University Press
6. Garfinkel PE, Garner DM, 1982. *Anorexia nervosa: a multidimensional perspective.* New York: Brunner/Mazel
7. Crisp AH, 1980. *Anorexia nervosa: let me be.* London: Academic Press
8. American Psychiatric Association, 1994. *Diagnostic and Statistical Manual of Mental Disorders (4th* ed). Washington, DC: APA
9. Kaye WH *et al*, 1987. Reduced cerebrospinal fluid levels of immunoreactive pro-opiomelanocortin related peptides (including beta-endorphin) in anorexia nervosa. *Life Sciences* 41:18, 2147-55
10. Gardner DM, Garfinkel PE (eds), 1985. *Handbook of psychotherapy for anorexia nervosa and bulimia.* New York: Guilford Press
11. Keys A *et al*, 1950. *The biology of human starvation.* Minneapolis: University of Minnesota Press
12. Wakeling A, 1985. Neurobiological aspects of feeding disorders. *Journal of Psychiatric Research* 19:191
13. Russell GFM, 1979. Bulimia nervosa: an ominous variant of anorexia nervosa. *Psychological Medicine* 9, 429
14. *Ibid*
15. Cooper PJ, Fairburn CG, 1983. Binge-eating and self-induced vomiting in the community: a preliminary study. *British Journal of Psychiatry* 142, 139
16. Kaye WH *et al*, 1990. CSF monoamine levels in normal-weight bulimia: evidence for abnormal noradrenergic activity. *American Journal of Psychiatry* 147:2, 225-29
17. Kaye WH *et al*, 2000. Effects of acute tryptophan depletion on mood in bulimia nervosa. *Biological Psychiatry* 47:2, 151-57
18. Pirke KM, 1996. Central and peripheral noradrenalin regulation in eating disorders. *Psychiatry Research* 62:1, 43-49
19. Kaye WH, Weltzin TE, 1991. Neurochemistry of bulimia nervosa. *Journal of Clinical Psychiatry* 52 (Suppl,) 21-8
20. Marrazzi MA *et al*, 1997. Endogenous codeine and morphine in anorexia and bulimia nervosa. *Life Sciences* 60:20, 1741-47
21. Kaye & Weltzin 1991, *op cit*
22. Hirschberg AL, 1998. Hormonal regulation of appetite and food intake. *Annals of Medicine* 30:1, 7-20
23. Kaye & Weltzin 1991, *op cit*

24. *Ibid*
25. Ill fitting genes: the biology of weight and shape control in relation to body composition and eating disorders [editorial]. *Psychological Medicine* 1997 27:3, 505-8

12. Dietetic treatments

1. Wardle J *et al*, 2000. Stress, dietary restraint and food intake. *Journal of Psychosomatic Research* 48:2, 195-202

13. Psychiatric therapy of depression, bulimia and anorexia

1. Robins LN, Locke BZ, Regier DA, 1991. An overview of psychiatric disorders in America. In Robins LN, Regier DA (eds), *Psychiatric Disorders in America: The Epidemiologic Catchment Area Study*. New York, NY: Free Press, 328-366
2. *Ibid*
3. Kessler RC, Zhao S, Blazer DG *et al*, 1997. Prevalence, correlates and course of minor depression and major depression in the National Comorbidity Survey. *Journal of Affective Disorders* 45, 19-30
4. Shelton RC, Davidson J, Yonkers K *et al*, 1997. The undertreatment of dysthymia. *Journal of Clinical Psychiatry* 58, 59-65
5. Simon GE, von Korff M, 1995. Recognition, management, and outcomes of depression in primary care. *Archives of Family Medicine* 4, 99-105
6. Keller MB, Klerman GL, Lavori PW *et al*, 1982. Treatment received by depressed patients. *Journal of the American Medical Association* 248, 1848-55
7. Goethe JW, Szarek BL, Cook WL,1988. A comparison of adequately vs inadequately treated depressed inpatients. *Journal of Nervous and Mental Disorders* 24, 75-80
8. Spitzer RL, Kroenke K, Linzer M, 1995. Health related quality of life in primary care patients with mental disorders: results from the PRIME-MD 1000 Study. *Journal of the American Medical Association* 274, 1511-17
9. Shelton RC, Davidson J, Yonkers K *et al*, 1997. The undertreatment of dysthymia. *Journal of Clinical Psychiatry* 58, 59-65
10. Greenberg PE, Stiglin LE, Finkelstein SN, 1993. The economic burden of depression in 1990. *Journal of Clinical Psychiatry* 54, 405-19
11. Shelton RC, Davidson J, Yonkers K *et al*, 1997. The undertreatment of dysthymia. *Journal of Clinical Psychiatry* 58, 59-65
12. Greenberg PE, Stiglin LE, Finkelstein SN, 1993. Depression: a neglected major illness. *Journal of Clinical Psychiatry* 54, 419-24
13. Schork EJ, Eckert ED, Halmi KA, 1994. The relationship between psychopathology, eating disorder diagnosis and clinical outcome at 10-year follow-up in anorexia nervosa. *Comprehensive Psychiatry* 35, 11
14. Keys A, Brozek J, Henschel A, 1950. *The Biology of Human Starvation*. Minneapolis: University of Minnesota Press
15. Collings S, King M, 1994. Ten-year follow-up on 50 patients with bulimia nervosa. *British Journal of Psychiatry* 164, 80-97
16. American Psychiatric Association, 1993. Practice Guideline for Eating Disorders. *American Journal of Psychiatry* 150, 212-28
17. Freeman CP, 1991. A practical guide to the treatment of of bulimia nervosa. *Journal of Psychosomatic Research* 35, 41-49
18. Wood A, 1993. Pharmacotherapy of bulimia nervosa – experience with fluoxetine. *International Clinical Psychopharmacology* 8, 295-99
19. Goldbloom DS, Olmsted MP, 1994. Pharmacotherapy with fluoxetine: assessment of clinically significant attitudinal change. *American Journal of Psychiatry* 150, 770-74

INDEX